Biological Activities of Pyrazole Scaffolds

Rajat Kalra
Archana Kapoor

Biological Activities of Pyrazole Scaffolds

LAP LAMBERT Academic Publishing

Imprint

Any brand names and product names mentioned in this book are subject to trademark, brand or patent protection and are trademarks or registered trademarks of their respective holders. The use of brand names, product names, common names, trade names, product descriptions etc. even without a particular marking in this work is in no way to be construed to mean that such names may be regarded as unrestricted in respect of trademark and brand protection legislation and could thus be used by anyone.

Cover image: www.ingimage.com

Publisher:
LAP LAMBERT Academic Publishing
is a trademark of
International Book Market Service Ltd., member of OmniScriptum Publishing Group
17 Meldrum Street, Beau Bassin 71504, Mauritius

Printed at: see last page
ISBN: 978-620-0-21421-8

Dr. Archana Kapoor M.
PHARM., PH. D
(Pharmaceutical Chemistry)
Assistant Professor
Department of Pharmaceutical
Sciences
Guru Jambheshwar Universty
of Science & Technology
Hisar, Haryana, India, 125001
archanarajpal06@gmail.com

Mr. Rajat Kalra M. PHARM
(Pharmaceutical Chemistry)
Assistant Professor
Department of Pharmaceutical
Sciences
Atam Institute of Pharmacy
Garhi/ Hansi, Haryana, India,
125033
rohillarajat@gmail.com

Preface

This book is going to be very helpful for the post graduate scholars and the research scholars at the beginning of their research carrier and will help them in selection of their research projects if based on pyrazole moiety.

This gives a brief outlook on the Pyrazole- a five membered heterocyclic ring and its importance from the chemistry as well as medicinal aspect. This includes general information, different synthetic procedures and medicinal activity of pyrazole bearing active compounds. The medicinal activity was described along with brief literature and the structure of the active compounds showing different biological activities *viz.,* antimicrobial, anticancer, antiviral, antimalarial, anti-inflammatory and analgesic activities. And while discussing the medicinal activity of different compounds containing pyrazole nucleus we have given the structures of starting materials as well as coloured representation of pathology of different diseases which makes this book a unique and different from others.

We hope our readers will find this book as an introductory tool for designing of new molecules and will be of widespread use further helping in learning and becoming a complete reference for the medicinal chemist.

Thanks for reading.

Contents

Chapter 1

Pyrazole

Abstract Pyrazole is five-membered and two nitrogen-containing heterocyclic compound and there are various methods for the synthesise of pyrazole. It is a part of azole family. Various noble pyrazole derivatives have been found that have the number of biological activities such as antimicrobial, antifungal, anticancer antiviral and much more. In this chapter, there is a brief introduction of pyrazole, its physical properties and synthethi procedures.

Keywords Pyrazole, Heterocyclic, Biological activities

1.1. Pyrazole

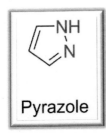

Pyrazole is five-membered heterocyclic compound in which two double and two adjacent nitrogen atoms are present. They are related to azole family with molecular formula $C_3H_4N_2$ [1] [2]. In 1889, first time pyrazole was achieved by Buchner on heating pyrazole-3,4,5-tricarboxylic acid at 230-240 °C [3]. Japanese scientist in 1954 identified first natural occurring pyrazole 3-N-nonylpyrazole from *Houttuynia cordata* (commomn name Dokudami in Japanese) a plant belonging to Saururaceae family and in 1959 pyrazolic amino acid: levo- β- (1 - pyrazolyl)alanine from seeds of water melon [4].

1.2. Tautomerism and Isomerism

Tautomerism is phenomena in which migration of protons takes place between the nitrogen atoms within the ring [5]. Pyrazole exhibited two identical tautomeric form. Speedy shifting of hydrogen atom from one nitrogen atom to another atom take place in pyrazole [6][7].

Tautomerism in Pyrazole

1.3. Physical Properties

The bond length between position 3 and 4 is longest bond with bond length of 1.416 A° and the ionization energy of pyrazole is about 9.15 eV [8].

Pyrazole

	Bond length (Å)	Bond angles (°)
Reference: *Gupta RR and Kumar M and Gupta V (1998) Heterocyclic Chemistry. Volume II: Five-Membered Heterocycles*	N_1-N_2= 1.349 N_2-C_3= 1.331 C_3-C_4= 1.416 C_4-C_5= 1.373 C_5-N_1= 1.359 N_1-H= 0.998	$C_5-N_1-N_2$= 113.1 $N_1-N_2-C_3$= 104.1 $N_2-C_3-C_4$= 111.9 $C_3-C_4-C_5$= 104.5 $C_4-C_5-N_1$= 104.1

Melting point (°C)	Boiling point (°C)	Log P	Dipole moment (μ, D)	Basic Pk$_{BH+}$ (proton acceptor)	Acid pKa In water (lose of protons)	UV (λmax nm, log ε)	IR (cm^{-1})	X-ray (CSD)
69-70	186-188 (58 mm of Hg)	0.1-0.26	1.92 (in benzene)	2.52	14.21	211 (3.49)	3524 (υ_{NH} gas)	PYRZOL

Table 1: Physical Properties of Pyrazole [10-14]

1.4. Synthesis of Pyrazoles

There are various methods to synthesize pyrazole, some are given below:

1.4.1. Knorr Pyrazole Synthesis

The synthesis of pyrazole was firstly noticed in 1883. This reaction also known as Knorr reaction. In this reaction hydrazine or substituted hydrazines reacted with 1,3-dicarbonyl or β dicarbonyl compounds to obtained the pyrazole or pyrazolone ring system. When hydrazine or substituted hydrazines reacted with symmetrical dicarbonyl compounds, it gives a single pyrazole isomer while unsymmetrically-substituted dicarbonyls compounds can give one or two isomers. When ketoesters treated with hydrazines or substituted hydrazines it can give pyrazolone ring system [15-17].

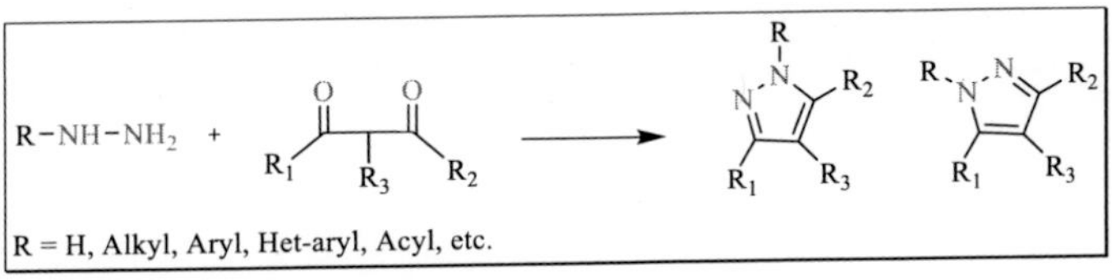

R = H, Alkyl, Aryl, Het-aryl, Acyl, etc.

1.4.2. Pechmann Pyrazole synthesis

In 1898, a German scientist Hans von Pechmann introduced pyrazole from Acetylene and diazomethane [20]

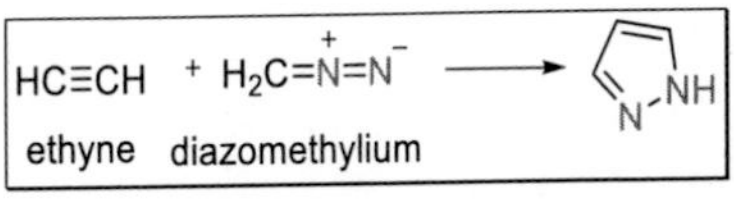

HC≡CH + $H_2C=N=N$ ⟶ pyrazole

ethyne diazomethylium

♣ Mechanisms for Pechmann Pyrazole synthesis [18-20]

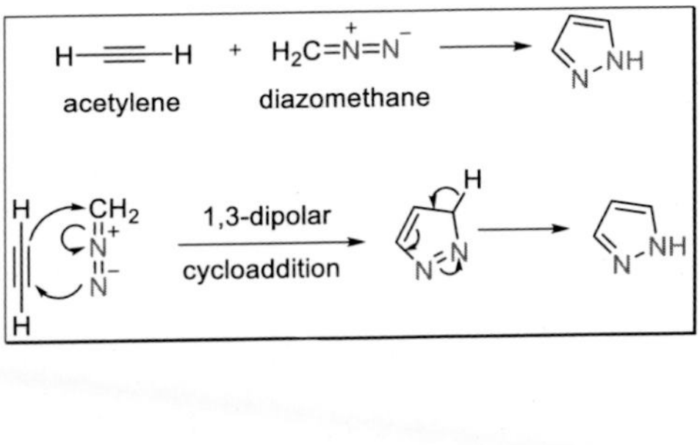

H———H + $H_2C=N=N$ ⟶

acetylene diazomethane

1,3-dipolar cycloaddition

3

1.5. Reactions of Pyrazole

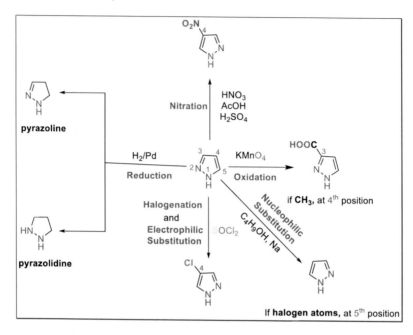

1.6. Biological Activities of Pyrazole

- Antimicrobial
- Anticancer
- Antiviral
- Analgesic and Anti-inflammatory
- Antimalarial Activity
- Anticonvulsant
- Herbicidal
- Antioxidant
- Antipyretic
- Antimycobacterial (T.B)

4

References

1. Builla JA, Vaquero JJ and Barluenga J (Eds) (2011) Modern Heterocyclic Chemistry (I^{st} Edn). Wiley-VCH Verlag GmbH & Co.KGaA

2. Kalra. R, Kumar S (2018) Synthesis and Antimicrobial Activity of 5-(Substituted-Phenyl)-3-(Furan-2-Yl)-4,5-Dihydro-1H-Pyrazole Compounds Using Silver Trifluro Methane Sulphonate as Catalyst. Der Pharmacia Lettre 10(8):57-67

3. Bansal R (1999) Heterocyclic Chemistry, (3rd edn), New age International Publisher

4. Wiley RH (Ed) (1967) Chemistry of Heterocyclic Compounds, Volume 22. John Wiley & Sons, Ltd

5. Schmidt A, Dreger A (2011) Recent Advances in the Chemistry of Pyrazoles. Properties, Biological Activities, and Syntheses".Current Organic Chemistry 15:1423. https://doi.org/10.2174/138527211795378263

6. Kornis, G. I. (2000) Pyrazoles, Pyrazolines, and Pyrazolones. Kirk-Othmer Encyclopedia of Chemical Technology. John Wiley & Sons

7. Joule JA, Mills K (2010) Heterocyclic Chemistry, (5th Edn). John Wiley & Sons, Ltd., Publication, p 485

8. Eicher T, Hauptmann S (2003) The Chemistry of Heterocycles Structure, Reactions, Syntheses and Applications. second Completely Revised, and Enlarged edn, Wiley-Vch Gmbh & Co. KGaA

9. Gupta RR et al (1999) Heterocyclic Chemistry, Volume ll: Five-MemberedHeterocycles. Springer-Verlag Berlin Heidelberg GmbH

10. Kumar S, Kalra R (2018) Valuable Heterocyclic Pyrazole. Lambert Academic Publishing

11. Koldobskii GI, Ostrovskii VA (1988) Acid-base properties of five-membered nitrogen-containing heterocycles (review). Chem Heterocycl Compd 24:469. https://doi.org/10.1007/BF00755683

12. Albert A et al (1948) The Strength of Heterocyclic Bases. J. Chem. 0:2240-2249, DOI: 10.1039/JR948000224

13. Serjeant EP, Dempsey B (1965) Dissociation Constants of Organic Acids and Bases in Aqueous, solution, Butterworths, London, 1965; Supplement, 1972.

14. Van Nostrand's Scientiþc Encyclopedia, Copyright © 2006 John Wiley & Sons, Inc.

15. Li Jack J (2014) Name Reactions A Collection of Detailed Mechanisms and Synthetic Applications, (5th Edn). Springer Int.Pub Switzerland

16. Hassner A, Stumer C (2002) Organic Syntheses Based on Name Reactions,(2nd Edn), vol 22. TETRAHEDRON Org.Chem. Series Elsevier

17. Li jack J (eds) (2005) Name Reactions In Heterocyclic Chemistry. A John Wiley & Sons, Inc., Publication

18. V Pechmann, H Duisberg CBer (1898) 31:2950.

19. Li jack J (2003) Name Reactions A Collection of Detailed Reaction Mechanisms, (2nd Edn). springer GmbH

20. Li jack J (2002) Name Reactions A Collection of Detailed Reaction Mechanisms, (1st Edn). springer GmbH

21. Wang Z (2010) Comprehensive Organic Name Reactions and Reagents. John Wiley & Sons, Inc

Chapter 2

Antimicrobial activity

Abstract The aim of this chapter is to provide focus on recent research work by various researchers on pyrazole derivatives which possess significant antimicrobial activity. There is a collection of literature work reported by various researchers on the anti-microbial activity of pyrazole. Antimicrobial are the drugs which used for the treatment and prevention of relapses of microbial infection. Antibiotic resistance is a great challenge in recent time. Morbidity and mortality rate are increased due to antibiotic resistance. Antimicrobial drugs are mostly daily prescribed drug.

Keywords Pyrazole, Heterocyclic, Antimicrobial activity

Introduction

The rate of morbidity and mortality is increased antibiotic resistance is current worldwide health issue due to excessive use of antimicrobial drugs. As result an effective, the discovery of new antimicrobial agent's appeal. The compound containing pyrazole nucleus exhibited various biological activities such as antimicrobial, anti-inflammatory, antiviral, antitumor activities and antimalarial. Pyrazole is five-membered heterocycles compounds which contain two neighbouring nitrogen atoms in their ring structure. Pyrazole associated with the group of azoles in which two double bonds are present with the molecular formula of $C_3H_4N_2$ [1-18]

(Hashem et al.) synthesized numbers of quinoline, chromene pyrazole derivatives (**scheme 1,2,3,4**) via using 7-Amino-3-phenyl-[1, 2, 4] triazolo [4, 3-*a*] pyrimidin-5(1*H*)-one (**I**) as key intermediate. It was noticed that compounds (**II-VI**) showed the most potent antimicrobial activity towards four strains (gram positive) *S. aureus* and *B. subtilis* and (gram negative) P. *aeruginosa*, *E. coli*, and *Salmonella typhi*. Authors also noticed that these active compounds also showed antifungal activity against *A. fumigatus*, *G. candidum*, *C. albicans*, and *S. racemosum* when Clotrimazole used as reference drug [11].

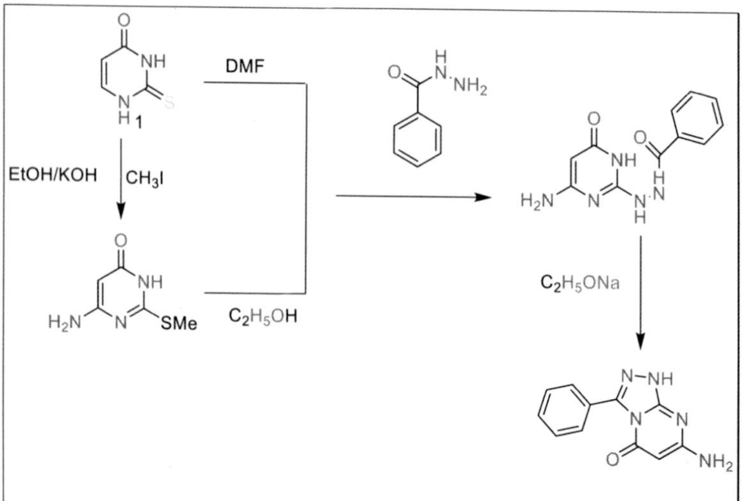

Synthesis of 7-Amino-3-phenyl-[1, 2, 4] triazolo [4, 3-*a*] pyrimidin-5(1*H*)-one

scheme 1

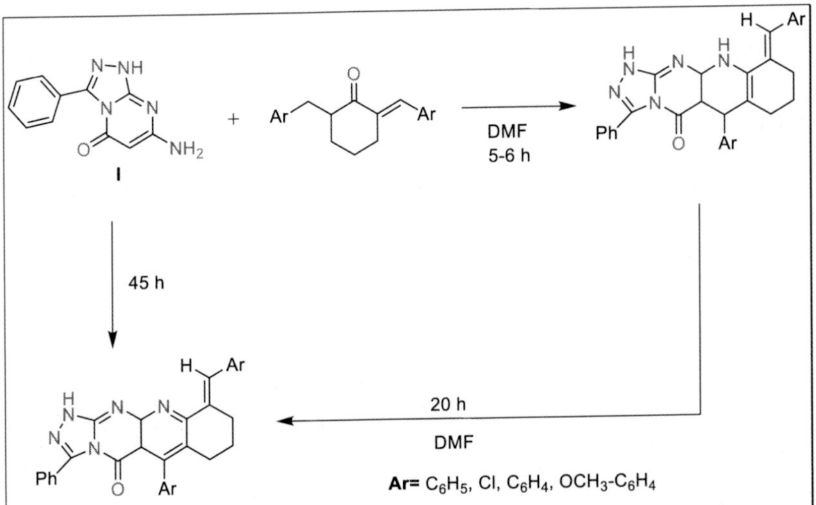

scheme 2
Synthesis of [1,2,4]triazolo[4',3':1,2]pyrimido[4,5-b]quinoline derivatives

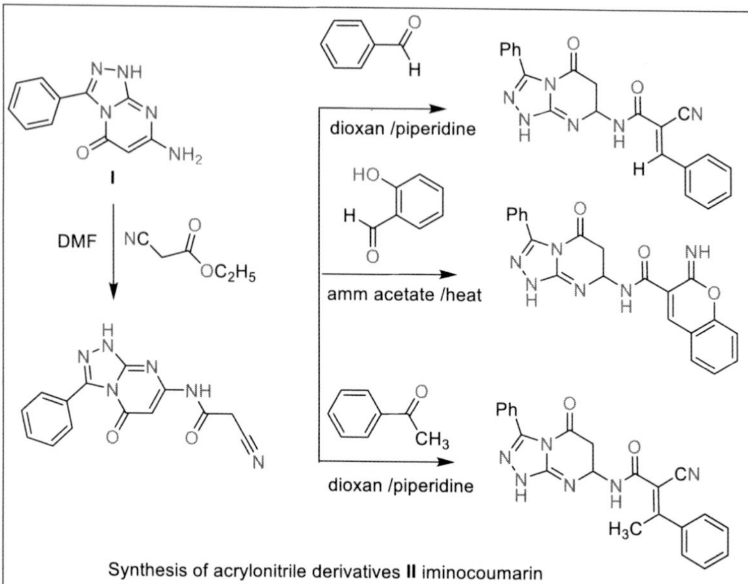

Synthesis of acrylonitrile derivatives **II** iminocoumarin

scheme 3

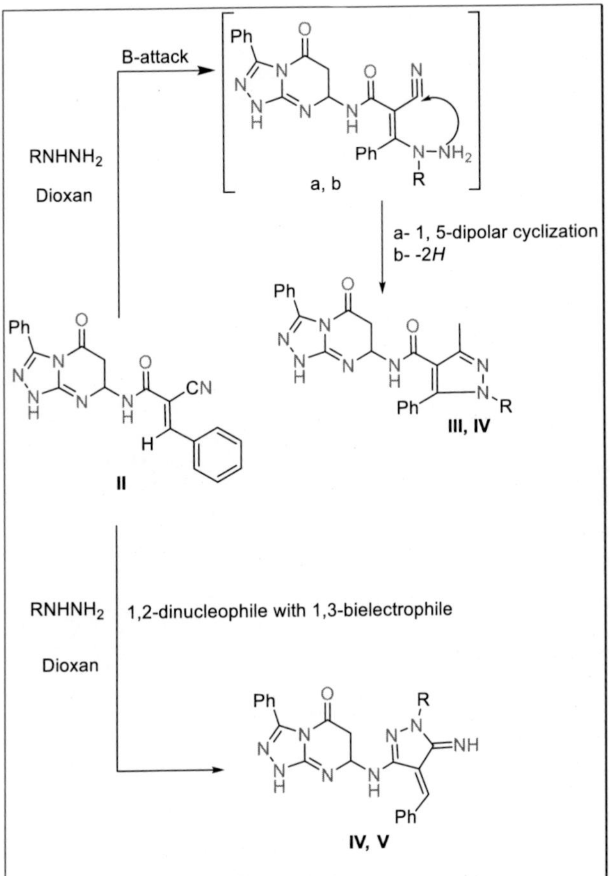

Synthesis of pyrazole derivatives

scheme 4

(Helal et al.) synthesized various 5-Aminopyrazole, Pyrazolo [1, 5-*a*] pyrimidine, bispyrazole and bispyridone derivatives which had antipyrinyl moiety (scheme 5, 6, 7) using 2-cyano-N-(1, 5-dimethyl-3-oxo-2-phenyl-2, 3-dihydro-1*H*-pyrazol-4-yl) acetamide as starting martial. An intermediate furnish 5-aminopyrazole (**VIII**) used as the key to prepare the more pyrazole derivatives. In conclusion, among the synthesized derivatives, three compound **VII** and **X** found to be most potent antimicrobial agents against gram-positive bacteria such as *Staphylococcus aureus*, *Bacillus subtilis*, *Enterococcus faecalis* and *Staphylococcus pyogenes*. On other hand, the compound **VII** found to be the most active towards gram-negative bacteria such as *Pseudomonas aeruginosa*, *Escherichia coli*, *Salmonella Typhimurium* and *Klebsiella pneumonia*. It was also noticed that the compounds **VII** and **X** possess excellent anti-fungal active towards *G. azeae* when Azithromycin and Ketoconazole used as reference drugs [12].

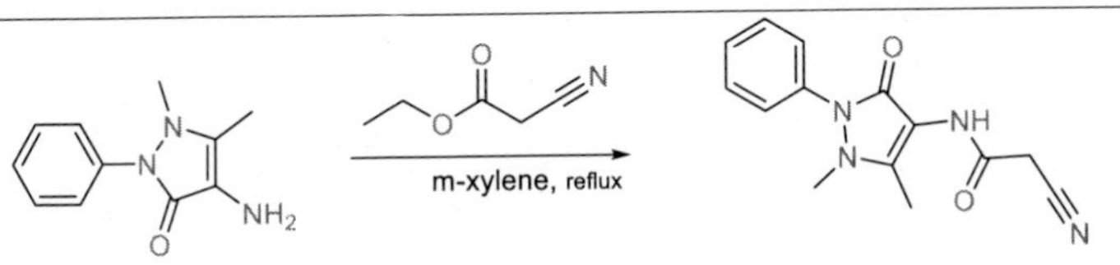

Synthesis of 2-cyano-N-(1,5-dimethyl-3-oxo-2-phenyl-2,3-dihydro1H-pyrazol-4-yl)acetamide

scheme 5

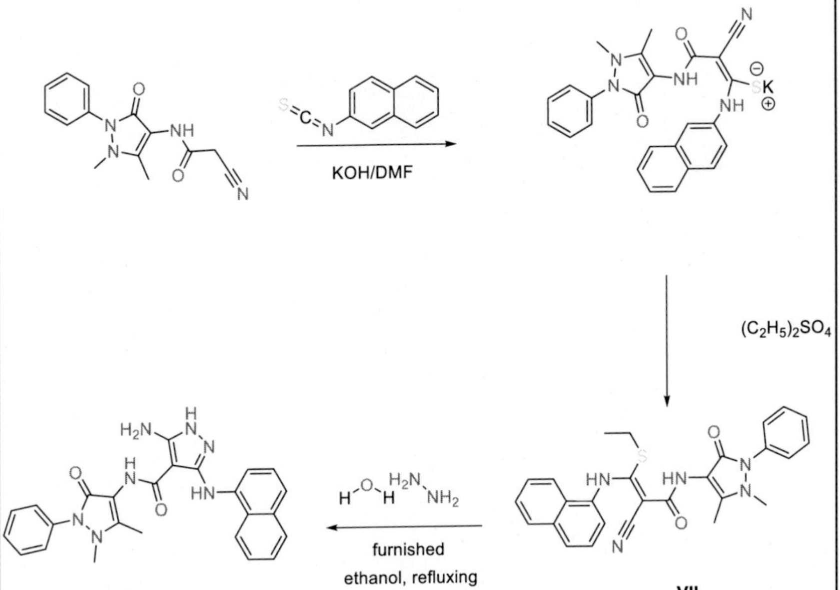

synthesis of 5-aminopyrazole derivative

scheme 6

(Refata et al.) synthesized number of novel hydrazide, pyrazole, triazine, isoxazole, and pyrimidine derivatives. All compounds were screened for their antimicrobial activity. Among the synthesized compounds, three products (**XI-XIV**) (**scheme** 7) possess the best anti-microbial activity against B. *subtilis* and E. *coli* bacterial strains. It was also concluded that all newly synthesized products showed very poor antifungal activity when Ampicillin and Clotrimazole used as reference drug [13].

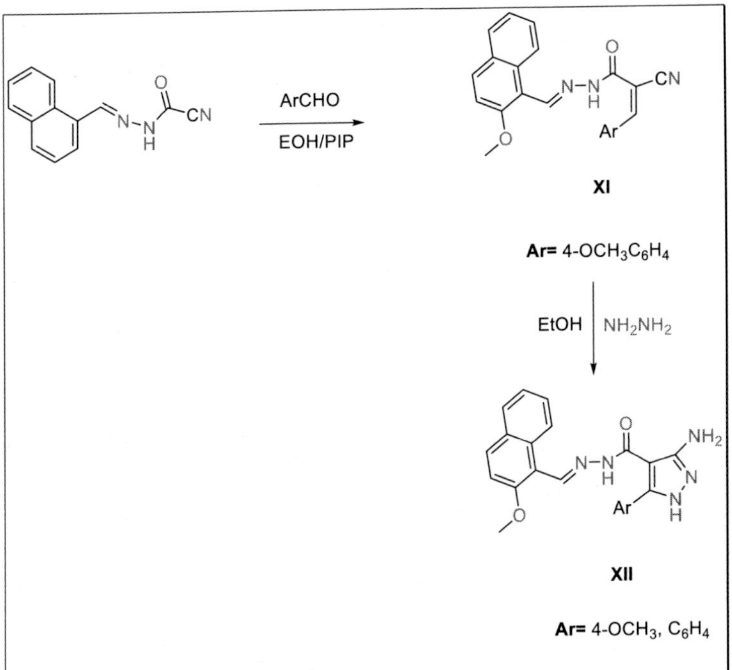

scheme 7

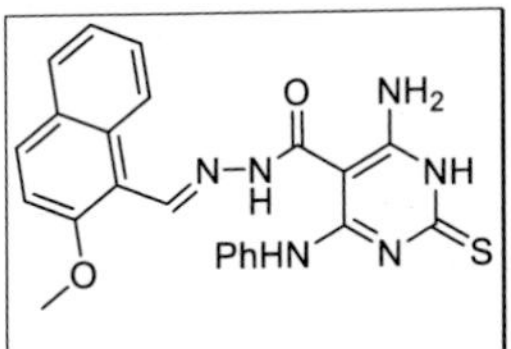

XIII

(Dhanapal et al.) synthesized number of 1, 2-dihydroquinoxaline-3-yl-3-substitutedphenyl-1*H*-pyrazole-4-Carbaldehyde pyrazole derivatives (scheme 8). The synthesized derivatives were screened for their antimicrobial activity. It was found that the compound **IV** showed excellent antimicrobial activity towards gram-positive bacterial strains i.e., *Staphylococcus aureus*, (ATCC) 914, B*acillus cereus* ATCC 11778 and gram-negative bacterial strains i.e., *Escherichia coli* ATCC 25922 and *Pseudomonas aeruginosa ATCC 2853.* Authors concluded that the pyrazole-4-carbaldehyde-incorporated quinoxaline was important for their antimicrobial activity [14].

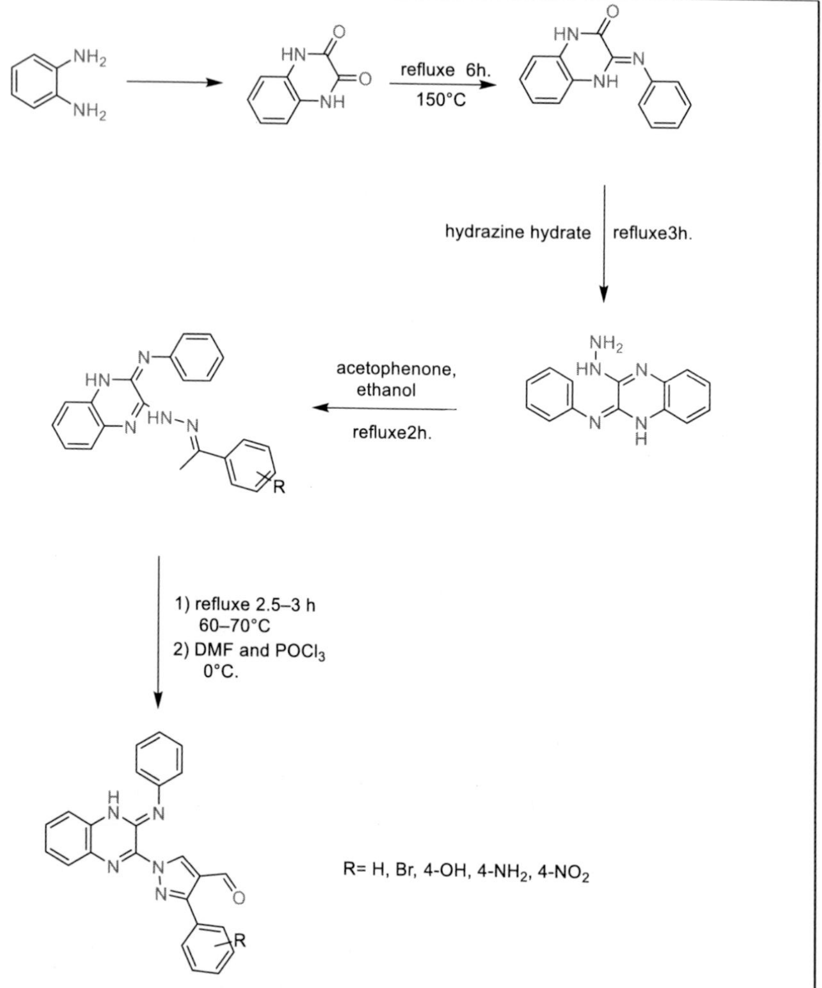

R= H, Br, 4-OH, 4-NH$_2$, 4-NO$_2$

XIV

scheme 8

R=

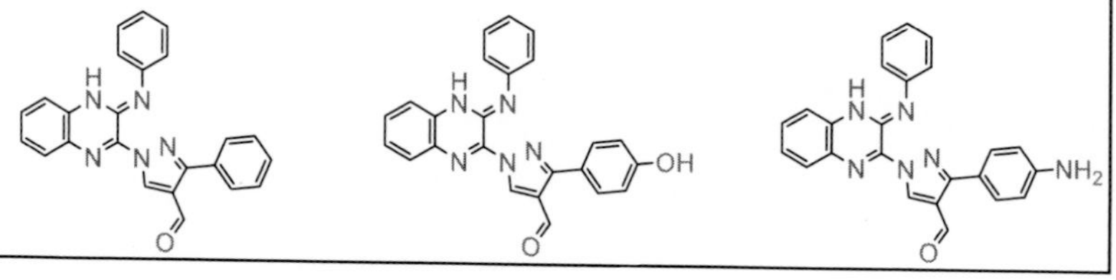

Via Vilsmeier Haack formylation and Hantzsch reaction novel thiazole substituted pyrazole derivatives (scheme **9, 10 ,11**) 1-[4-(2,3,4-substituted-phenyl)thiazol-2-yl]-3-(2,3,4-substituted-phenyl)-1*H*pyrazole-4-carbaldehyde (4a–m), 4-[4-(4-substituted-phenyl) thiazol-2-yl]-3-(4-substituted-phenyl)-1-phenyl-1*H*-pyrazole (**XVIa–i**), 4-[4-(4-substituted phenyl)thiazol-2-yl]-1-phenyl-1*H*-pyrazol-3-amine (**XVIIa–g**) were reported by (Gaikwad et al.) All newly reported compounds were screened for their antimicrobial activity. It was noticed that most of the compounds showed good antimicrobial activity against both gram-positive and gram-negative bacterial strains i.e., *Bacillus subtilis* (2250), *Staphylococcus aureus* (2079), *Escherichia coli* (2109), and *Pseudomonas aeruginosa* (2036). It was also observed that the newly prepared compounds also possess superior antifungal activity towards two fungi stains of *Candida albicans* (3471) and *Aspergillus niger* (545) and Nystatin used as reference drug [15].

scheme 9

Compounds	R₁	R₂	R₃	R₄	R₅	R₆
XVa	H	H	H	H	Br	H
XVb	CF₃	H	CF₃	F	OMe	H
XVc	H	Br	H	H	NO₂	H
XVd	CF₃	H	CF₃	NO₂	H	H
XVe	H	NO₂	H	F	OMe	H
XVf	H	NO₂	H	H	Br	H
XVg	H	NO₂	H	CF₃	H	CF₃
XVh	CF₃	H	CF₃	CF₃	H	CF₃
XVi	H	Br	H	H	Br	H
XVj	CF₃	H	CF₃	H	Br	H
XVk	CF₃	H	CF₃	H	Cl	H
XVl	H	Br	H	H	Cl	H
XVm	H	Cl	H	H	NO₂	H

17

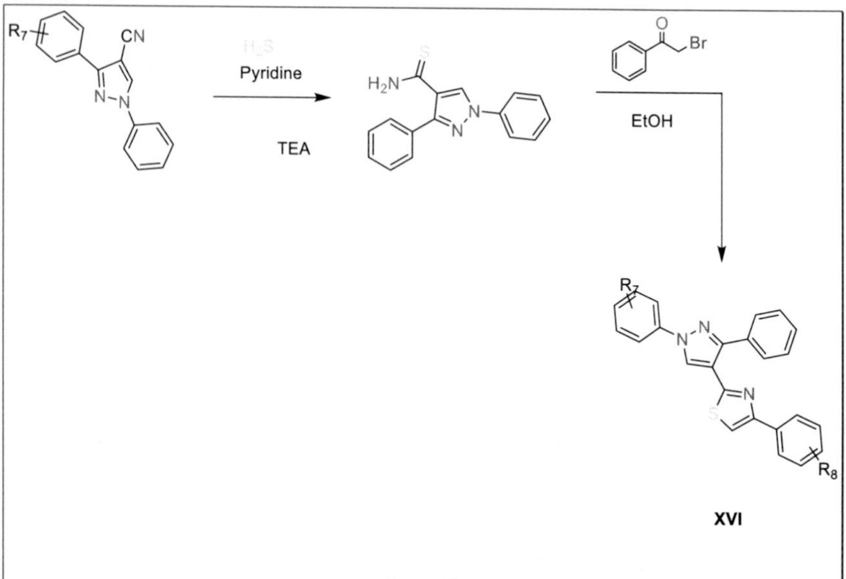

scheme 10

Compounds	R₇	R₈
XVIa	F	NO_2
XVIb	F	Cl
XVIc	F	H
XVId	F	Br
XVIe	F	F
XVIf	F	CH_3
XVIg	Br	CH_3
XVIh	Br	NO_2
XVIi	Br	H

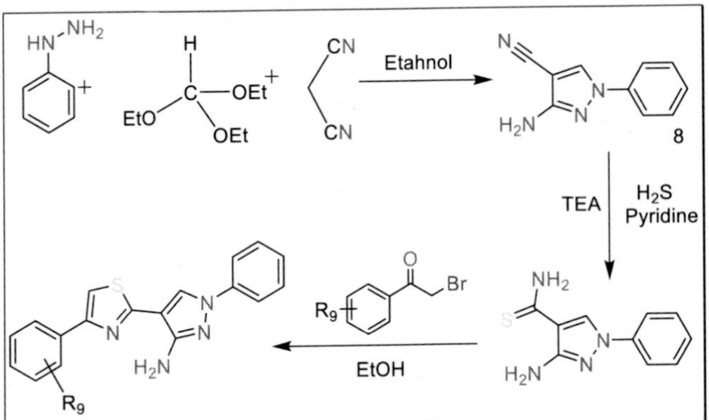

scheme 11

XVII

Compounds	R₉
XVIIa	F
XVIIb	Cl
XVIIc	Br
XVIId	CH₃
XVIIe	H
XVIIf	4NO₂
XVIIg	3 NO₂

References

1. Kumar, Sunil, K Rajat. 2018. "Synthesis and Antimicrobial Activity of 5- (Substituted-Phenyl) -3- (Furan-2- Yl) -4, 5-Dihydro-1H-Pyrazole Compounds Using Silver Trifluro Methane Sulphonate as Catalyst." 2(2): 57–67.
2. Khloya, P., 2013. "Synthesis of some novel 4-arylidene pyrazoles as potential antimicrobial agents". Organic and Medicinal Chemistry Letters. 3:9.
3. Amir M, et al. Synthesis and antimicrobial activity of pyrazolinones and pyrazoles having benzothiazole moiety. Med Chem Res. 2012. 21: 1261.
4. Madhava, R., et al. Synthesis and antimicrobial activity of some novel pyrazoles. Der Pharmacia Lettre. 2012. 4: 1123-1128.
5. Fatima A, et al. Design, Synthesis, antimicrobial and anti-inflammatory activity of N-pyrazolyl benzamide derivatives.
6. Med chem, 2015. 5: 521-527.
7. Mor, S., et al. Med Chem Res. 2012. 21: 3541.
8. Jayanna, ND., et al. Synthesis and biological evaluation of novel 5,7-dichloro-1,3-benzoxazole derivatives. Med Chem Res. 2013. 22: 5814.
9. Abd-El, G., et al. Med Chem Res. 2012; 21: 98.
10. Kumar P, et al. Synthesis and biological evaluation of some pyrazole derivativesas anti-inflammatory–antibacterial agents. Med Chem Res. 2012. 21: 3396.
11. Rashad AA, et al. Design, synthesis and preliminary antiviral screening ofnew N-phenylpyrazole and dihydroisoxazole derivatives. Med Chem Res. 2010. 19: 1025.
12. Tantawy AS, et al. Synthesis and antiviral activity of new 3-methyl-1, 5-diphenyl-1H-pyrazole derivatives. Med Chem Res. 2012. 21: 4139.
13. Prasad R. Sujay M, et al. 2017 'Anticancer Activity of Iridium (III) Complexes Based on a Pyrazole-Appended QuinolineBased BODIPY". Inorg. Chem. 56(2): 12232-12247.
14. Hura, N., et al. 2018 "Drug-clinical agent molecular hybrid: Synthesis of diaryl(trifluoromethyl)pyrazoles as tubulin targeting anticancer agents". ACS Omega. 3 (2): 1955-1969.
15. Gouhar, SR., et al. 2013 "Synthesis and anticancer screening of some novel substituted pyrazole derivatives". Der Pharma Chemica.. 5(6):225-233
16. Tuha, A., 2008 "Synthesis and biological screening of some pyrazole derivatives as antimalarial and anti-leishmanial agents. A thesis submitted to the School of Graduate Studies of Addis Ababa University in partial fulfillment of the requirements for the Degree of Master of Science in Medicinal Chemistry". 32.
17. Verma M, et al. 2008 "Synthesis of some substituted pyrazole derivatives and their evaluation as antiprotozoal agents". Int. J. Chem. Sci. 6 (1): 179-184.
18. Builla-AJ., et al. 2011 "Modern Heterocyclic Chemistry". First Edition, Wiley-VCH Verlag GmbH & Co. KGaA, 1-9.
19. Pyrazole Encyclopædia Britannica, inc, https://www.britannica. com/science/pyrazole (2018)
20. Gouda, M A. et al. 2016. "Synthesis and Antimicrobial Activity of Some Novel Quinoline, Chromene , Pyrazole Derivatives Bearing Triazolopyrimidine Moiety." 5(5).
21. Helal, Mohamed Hamdy, Mohamed A. Salem, and Hala Mohamed Aly. 2017. "Synthesis, Antimicrobial Activity and Molecular Modeling of Some Novel 5-Aminopyrazole,

Pyrazolo[1,5-a]Pyrimidine, Bispyrazole and Bispyridone Derivatives Containing Antipyrinyl Moiety." Journal of Heterocyclic Chemistry 54(5): 2614–26.

22. Refat, Hala, and A Fadda. 2015. "Synthesis and Antimicrobial Activity of Some Novel Hydrazide, Pyrazole, Triazine, Isoxazole, and Pyrimidine Derivatives.doi 10.1002/jhet.2369

23. Visagaperumal Dhanapal, et al. 2016. "Synthesis, Characterization and Antimicrobial Activity of 1,2- Dihydroquinoxaline-3-Yl-3-Substitutedphenyl-1H-Pyrazole-4-Carbaldehyde." J. Heterocyclic Chem., 954–59. doi 10.1002/jhet.2663

24. Yildirir, Yilmaz. et al. 2010. "Synthesis and Antimicrobial Activity of Novel Thiazole Substituted Pyrazole Derivatives." (May): 954–59.

Chapter 3

Anticancer Activity

Abstract Cancer is a disease when cells lose the ability of control, growth, division and spread. As a result, there is a formation of a solid mass known as tumor and death is the end result of this disease. Cancer cells have the ability to spread to other body sites. There are various types of cancers reported. In India, Breast cancer is becoming a great challenge nowadays. The aim of this chapter is to provide focus on recent research work carried out by various researchers on pyrazole derivatives which possess significant anticancer activity.

Keywords Pyrazole, Heterocyclic, Anticancer activity

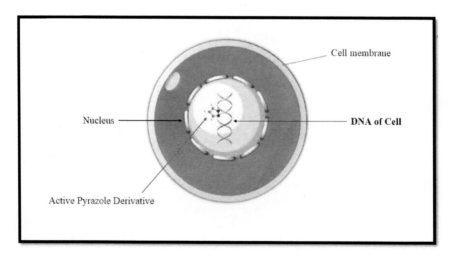

Fig 3.1. Pyrazole deraivatives cause death of cancer cell

Cancer is concerted described as a group of diseases which lose the control over growth, division, and spread of a group of cells, leading to a solid mass of cells termed as a tumor that infect and destroys adjoining tissues. The initial tumor, recognized as the primary tumor. The primary tumor is the most common causes of death due to spread in other body sites (by metastasis process) [1] [2]. There are various types of cancer such as Breast cancer [3], Lung cancer [4], Bladder cancer [5], Kidney cancer [6], Leukaemia [7] etc. Breast cancer is the most common cancer in India [8].

Pyrazole and its derivatives possessed anticancer activity [9] [10]. In this chapter, there is a collection of literature work reported by various researchers on the anticancer activity of pyrazole.

Some novel 1-cyanoacetyl-3,5-dimethylpyrazole derivatives were reported by (Metwally et al.) via using 3-(3,5-dimethyl-1*H*-pyrazol-1-yl)-3-oxopropanenitrile as starting material. All freshly prepared products were screened for their anticancer activity towards hepatocarcinoma cell line (HEPG2) and human breast adenocarcinoma cell line (MCF7) in the Sulphorodamine-B (SRB) assay method. Amongst synthesized derivatives two compounds **i** and **ii** found to be the most potent products of this series [11].

Ar = C_6H_5, 4-ClC_6H_4, 4-$NO_2C_6H_4$ R= H, Me, Cl

Novel pyrazole-5-carboxamide and pyrazole pyrimidine derivatives were produced by (Bo et al.). The synthesized compounds were screened for their anticancer activity against MGC-803 cell line. It was noticed that a compound **iii** found to be the most potent compound of this series and to prohibit the MGC-803 cell proliferation [12].

iii

(Ahmed et al.) prepared novel series of quinazolin-4-one derivatives linked to thiazolidinone, oxadiazole or pyrazole derivatives. All novel reported products were tested for anticancer activity towards MCF-7 breast cancer cell line when Doxorubicin used as standard drug. Amongst to all newly synthesized compounds, two products **iv** and **v** found to be the most active product of this series [13].

(Siddiqui et al.)reported a new series of steroidal oxadiazole, pyrrole, and pyrazole derivatives. All freshly prepared candidates were tested for their anticancer activity against human leukemia cell line (HL-60) in MTT assay method. The most active compound of this series was compound **vi** among to synthesized compounds [14].

vi

Novel steroidal pyrazolines derivatives were introduced by (Khanam et al.) All newly introduced synthesized cell lines. During MTT assay, it was found that compound **vii** possessed most potent anticancer as well as antimicrobial activity [15].

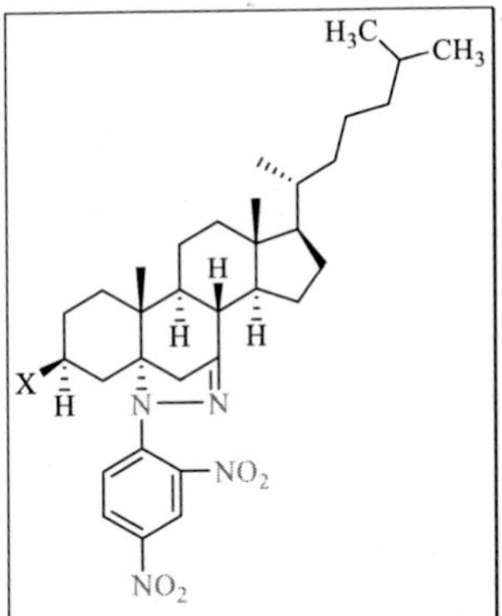

vii

X= Cl, H

(Park et al.) produced a new series of pyrazole oxime ether derivatives. All newly preapred products were screened for their anticancer activity against various cancer cell lines i.e., HepG2 (liver), MCF7 (breast), MKN45 (stomach), and A549 (lung). During SBR assay, it was found that the compound **viii** possessed the significant anticancer activity when Doxorubicin used as standard drug [16].

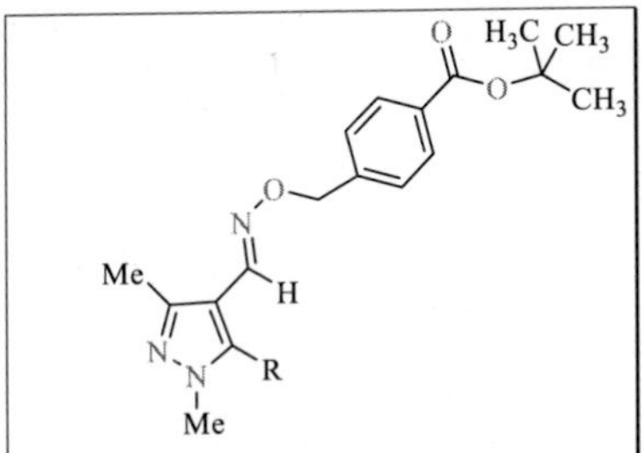

viii

R=

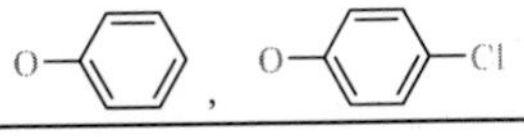

References

1. Avendano C, Menendez JC. (2008). Medicinal Chemistry of Anticancer Drugs. Elsevier ISBN: 978-0-444-52824-7
2. Thurston DE, Thurston DE. (2006). Chemistry and Pharmacology of Anticancer Drugs. CRC Press. Taylor & Francis
3. Clark A, Fallowfield L. (1991). Breast Cancer. London: CRC Press, https://doi.org/10.1201/9781482267563
4. Taylor C et al. (2017). Estimating the Risks of Breast Cancer Radiotherapy: Evidence from Modern Radiation Doses to the Lungs and Heart and from Previous Randomized Trials. Journal of Clinical Oncology 35:1641-1649. DOI: 10.1200/JCO.2016.72.0722
5. Droller, Michael J. (Eds) (2001) Bladder Cancer: Current Diagnosis and Treatment. Current Clinical Urology Humana Press. DOI: 10.1007/978-1-59259-097-1
6. Pfaffenroth EC, W Marston Linehan (2008) Genetic basis for kidney cancer: opportunity for disease-specific approaches to therapy, Expert Opinion on Biological Therapy 8(6):779-790. DOI: 10.1517/14712598.8.6.779
7. Galton DAG (1992) Haematological Differences Between Chronic Granulocytic Leukaemia, Atypical Chronic Myeloid Leukaemia, and Chronic Myelomonocytic Leukaemia, Leukemia & Lymphoma 7(5-6):343-350. DOI: 10.3109/10428199209049789
8. Gupta A et al (2015) A review of breast cancer awareness among women in India: Cancer literate or awareness deficit?.European Journal of Cancer 51:2058– 2066. http://dx.doi.org/10.1016/j.ejca.2015.07.008
9. Czarnomysy R et al (2018) A novel series of pyrazole-platinum (II) complexes as potential anti-cancer agents that induce cell cycle arrest and apoptosis in breast cancer cells. Journal of Enzyme Inhibition and Medicinal Chemistry 33(1):1006-1023. DOI: 10.1080/14756366.2018.1471687
10. Abdel-Aziz M, Gamal-Eldeen AM (2009) Synthesis and screening of anti-cancer, antioxidant, and anti-inflammatory activities of novel galloyl pyrazoline derivatives. Pharmaceutical Biology 47(9):854-863. DOI: 10.1080/13880200902946452
11. Ahmed, Marwa F., et al. CHEMISTRY Design, Synthesis, Molecular Modeling and Anti-Breast Cancer Activity of Novel Quinazolin-4-One Derivatives Linked to Thiazolidinone , Oxadiazole or Pyrazole Moieties. 2015, doi:10.1007/s00044-015-1357-1.
12. Bo, Jing, et al. "European Journal of Medicinal Chemistry Novel Pyrazole-5-Carboxamide and Pyrazole e Pyrimidine Derivatives: Synthesis and Anticancer Activity." European Journal of Medicinal Chemistry, vol. 90, Elsevier Masson SAS, 2015, pp. 889–96, doi:10.1016/j.ejmech.2014.12.013.
13. Khanam, Hena, et al. "Synthesis, Characterization, Antimicrobial and Anticancer Studies of New Steroidal Pyrazolines." Journal Of Saudi Chemical Society, King Saud University, 2012, doi:10.1016/j.jscs.2012.05.004.
14. Metwally, Nadia H., et al. "Synthesis and Anticancer Activity of Some New Heterocyclic Compounds Based on 1-Cyanoacetyl-3,5-Dimethylpyrazole." Research on Chemical Intermediates, Springer Netherlands, 2015, doi:10.1007/s11164-015-2074-6.
15. Park, Hyun-ja, et al. Identification of Antitumor Activity of Pyrazole Oxime Ethers. Vol. 15, 2005, pp. 3307–12, doi:10.1016/j.bmcl.2005.03.082.
16. Siddiqui, Tabassum, et al. "Synthesis, Characterization and Anticancer Studies of New Steroidal Oxadiazole, Pyrrole and Pyrazole Derivatives." Journal Of Saudi Chemical Society, King Saud University, 2012, doi:10.1016/j.jscs.2012.04.009

Chapter 4

Anti-Inflammatory and Analgesic Activities

Abstract The aim of this chapter is to provide focus on recent research work by various researchers on pyrazole derivatives which possess significant anti-inflammatory and analgesic effects. There is a collection of literature work reported by various researchers on the anti-inflammatory and analgesic activity of pyrazole. Prostaglandins are main mediators of inflammation and they are produced with prostanoids during metabolism of the arachidonic acid. Cyclooxygenase (COX) is an enzyme which catalyze arachidonic acid into prostaglandin H2. This enzyme has two isoforms (COX-1) and (COX-2). When COX-2 is overexpressed at the spot of injury they cause inflammation and pain at the injury site. NSAIDs decrease the biosynthesis of prostaglandins. The anti-inflammatory and analgesic effects of NSAIDs are associated with inhibition of the COX-2 enzyme.

Keywords Pyrazole, Heterocyclic, anti-inflammatory and analgesic activity

Introduction

Prostaglandins are the endogenous substance and the main potent negotiator of inflammation which take part in numerous physiological processes. These proteinoids are produced during metabolism of the arachidonic acid, prostaglandins are also produced with them. The oxidative transformation of arachidonic acid into prostaglandin H_2 is catalysed by an enzyme cyclooxygenase (COX). The enzyme (COX) occurs in two isoforms COX-1 and COX-2 [1-4]. The COX-1 isoform found in blood platelets, kidneys, and in the gastrointestinal tract while the COX-2 isoform is an inducible enzyme which is released when the various cells expressed to cytokines, mitogens and endotoxins during injury [5-6]. The main reason of inflammation and pain is that the enzyme COX-2 is overexpressed at the spot of injury site [6]. Mostly the non-steroidal anti-inflammatory drugs (NSAIDs) inhibition the transformation of arachidonic acid into prostaglandin H_2 biosynthesis COX reaction [7]. The anti-inflammatory and analgesic activity of NSAIDs are due to the inhibition of the COX-2 enzyme while on another hand, gastrointestinal irritation and ulcerative activity of NSAIDs due to the inhibition of the COX-1 enzyme [8].

Pyrazole and its derivatives possess the anti-inflammatory and analgesic activity [9]. In this chapter, there is a collection of literature work reported by various researchers on the anti-inflammatory and analgesic activity of pyrazole.

(Selvan et.) prepared a novel series of 1-(4-substitutedphenyl)-3-phenyl-1*H*-pyrazole-4-carbaldehydes via Vilsmeier-Haack reagent. All newly prepared compounds were screened for their anti-inflammatory and analgesic activities by using carrageenan-induced paw edema method and by the tail-flick method in Wistar albino mice. Among all compounds, compounds **I** showed the best anti-inflammatory as well as analgesic activity when compared to reference drug Diclofenac sodium [10].

I

R_1= F, Br, Cl

A new series contained *N*-phenyl-1-*H*-pirazoles and1,3,4-oxadiazole-2(3*H*)-thione was synthesized by (Costa et al.) All the prepared compounds were screened for their antinociceptive and *in-vivo* anti-inflammatory activity by using carrageenan-induced paw edema method in rats. In conclusion, three compounds **(II, LQFM-146)**, **(III, LQFM-147)** and **(IV, LQFM-148)** of this series found to be the most potent products due to the reduction of pro-inflammatory cytokines and they also inhibited an enzyme myeloperoxidas at doses 89, 178 and 356 mmol/kg p.o [11].

II	**III**	**IV**

(Lavanya et al.) synthesized some novel 1,3,4-thiadiazoles containing pyrazole and pyrrole nucleus derivatives via taking 1,3,4-thiadiazolacrylamides (**V**) as key intermediate. All the synthesized compounds were evaluated for their anti-inflammatory activity by using carrageenan-induced acute paw edema method in Wistar albino rats and found that seven compounds possessed anti-inflammatory activity but the compounds (**VI**) and (**VII**) possessed the most superior anti-inflammatory activity of this series when compared to reference drug Indomethacin [12].

V	**VI**	**VII**

R= C_6H_5, 4-Br-C_6H_4, 4-NO_2-C_6H_4, 4F--C_6H_4, 4-I--C_6H_4, 4-Cl--C_6H_4

R= NO_2, F

(Mandour et al.) prepared some novel 4,6-dimethoxy-5-(heterocycle)benzofuran derivatives via reaction of 1-(4,6-dimethoxybenzofuran-5-yl)ethenone (**VIII**) and its hydrazone derivatives (**IX**). All newly prepared compounds were evaluated for their anti-inflammatory, analgesic and anticonvulsant by using carrageenan-induced rat paw oedema method in adult male albino rats. In conclusion, among the synthesized compounds, (**X**) found to be most potent compound of this series when Flufenamic acid and Indomethacin used as reference drug [13].

| VIII | IX | X |

(Dhingra et al.) prepared novel *o*-Propargylated-N-acetylpyrazole derivative via using 1,3-Diarylpropenones **(XI)** as starting material. All newly prepared compounds were screened for their *in-vivo* anti-inflammatory activity by using the carrageenan-induced paw oedema model in rats. Amongst to all those compounds, compound **XII** and **XIII** exhibited the most promising anti-inflammatory activity as compared to standard drug Indomethacin [14].

| XI | XII | XIII |

$R_1 = R_3 = H$ $R_2 = H, Br, NO_2$

(Kuo et al.) introduced a novel series of 3,4-Dimethylpyrano[2,3-*c*]pyrazol-6-one derivatives. All freshly prepared products were evaluated for their analgesic and anti-inflammatory activities by using carrageenan-induced paw edema method in rats, and found that compounds, **XIV** and **XV** were the most potent compounds of this series when compared to standard drug Aminopyrine [15].

| XIV | XV |

R= CH_3

Some novel1,3,4-trisubstituted pyrazoles derivatives were prepared by [Georgey et al.] All newly synthesized compounds were tested for their anti-inflammatory and analgesic activities using carrageenan-induced rat paw edema model. In conclusion, among the synthesized

30

compounds, **XVI** possessed the most potent anti-inflammatory as well as analgesic activity when Phenylbutazone used as a standard drug [16].

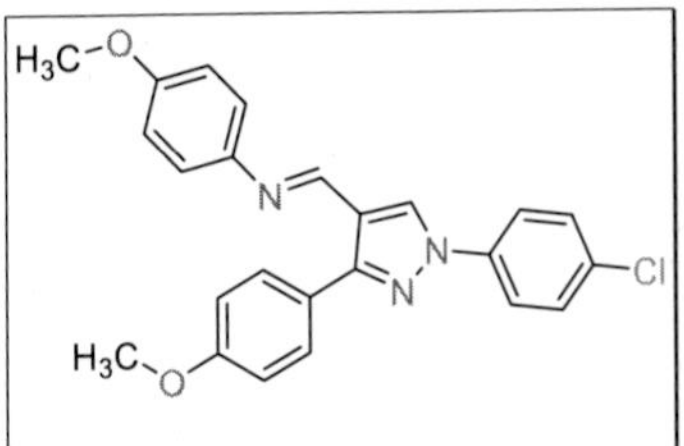

XVI

A new series of 1-(4-substituted phenyl)-3-phenyl-1*H*-pyrazole-4-carbaldehydes were prepared by (Selvam et al.) All newly prepared compounds were screened for their anti-inflammatory and analgesic activities by using carrageenan-induced paw edema method and by the tail-flick method in Wistar albino mice. Among all novel synthesized compounds, **XVII** possess the most potent anti-inflammatory as well as analgesic activities [17].

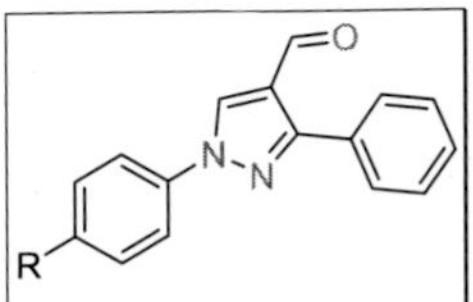

XVII

R= F, Br, Cl

Some novel pyrazole derivatives were prepared by (Kumar et al.) All freshly preapred compounds were screened for their antibacterial (*in-vitro*) and anti-inflammatory activity (*in-vivo*). During carrageenan-induced rat paw edema model, it was found that most of the compounds exhibited better anti-inflammatory as well as antibacterial activities but compound **XVIII** found to be the most potent compound of this series when compared to Indomethacin as reference drug [18].

XVIII

R= H, F, Cl, OCH₃   **R₁= Cl, CH₃**

A novel series of 1-Phenyl-3-(thiophen-2-yl)-1H-pyrazole-4-carbaldehyde were introduced by (Bakr et al.) All newly prepared compounds were evaluated for their antimicrobial, anti-inflammatory, and analgesic activities. Most of the compounds showed both analgesic and anti-inflammatory activities but in carrageenan-induced paw edema model and writhing assay, it was found that compounds **XIX** and **XX** possessed excellent anti-inflammatory, as well as analgesic activity as compared to standard drug Diclofenac sodium. It was also noticed that compound **XIX** was active against *Staphylococcus aureus* and *Enterobacter Cloaca* bacterial strains [19].

XIX   **XX**

Some new compounds were synthesized by (Domiati et al.) and were evaluated for their anti-inflammatory and analgesic activities by using carrageenan-induced rat paw edema model. The authors noticed that the compound **XXI** showed very high analgesic as well as anti-inflammatory activity than standard drug Indomethacin and Celecoxib. But it was found that compound was not the safest compound as it was causing ulcer in the stomach of the mice. In conclusion, among the synthesized compounds, two derivatives, compound **XXII** and compound **XXIII** possessed the safest clinical uses for analgesic and anti-inflammatory activities [20].

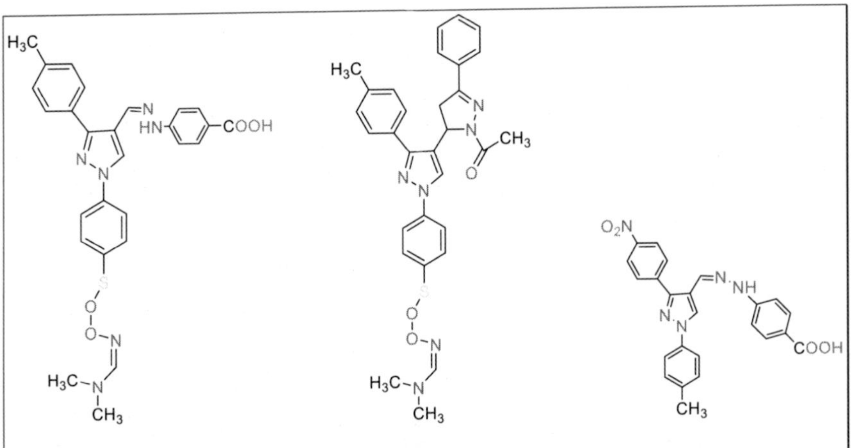

XXI   XXII   XXIII

(Kov et al.) reported novel 1,2,3-Triketone 2-(antipyrin-4-yl)hydrazones via azo-coupling reaction of 1,3-diketones **(XXIV)**. All newly prepared compounds were screened for their antipyretic and analgesic activities by taken Analgin as standard drug. It was found that the compound **XXVI** showed best analgesic activity but do not possess antipyretic activity while the compound **XXVI, (R= Ph)** possessed most potent antipyretic activity [21].

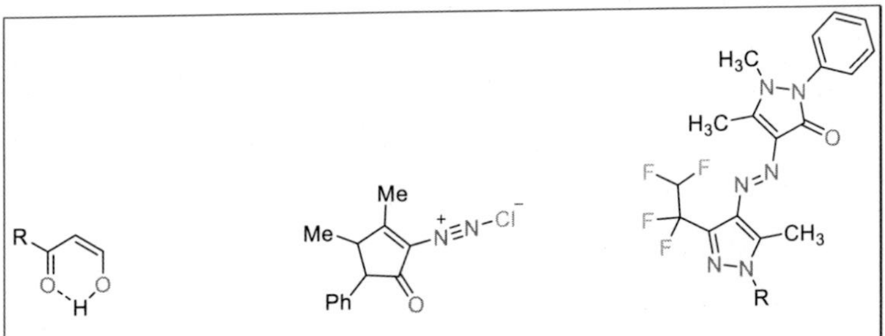

XXIV   XXV   XXVI

R= Me, H(CF$_2$)$_2$ R= (CH$_2$)$_2$OH, Ph

Novel pyrazole derivatives were synthesized by (Nagwa et al.) All newly synthesized compounds were screened for their anti-inflammatory and analgesic activities in carrageenan-induced rat paw edema method and p-benzoquinone-induced writhing test in mice. During the SAR (structural activity relationship) study, it was found that aryl moiety in pyrazole ring is important for the activity. In conclusion, it was found to be the compounds **XXVII** and **XXVIII** possessed the most potent analgesic and anti-inflammatory activities. On other hand, the

33

compound **XXIX** showed only analgesic activity when compared to standard drug Ibuprofen and Celecoxib [22].

| XXVII | XXVIII | XXIX |

(Jayanna et al.) [23] reported a novel series of 1-(5,7-dichloro-1,3-benzoxazol-2-yl)-3-phenyl-1*H*-pyrazole-4-carbaldehyde derivatives via condensation of 5,7-dichloro-2-hydrazino-1,3-benzoxazole **(XXX)** with various aromatic acetophenones **XXXI** in presence of methanol **XXXII**. All newly synthesized compounds were evaluated for their *in-vivo* antimicrobial as well as analgesic activities using acetic acid- induced writhing method in mice. In conclusion, among the synthesized compounds, compound **XXXIII** possessed the most promising analgesic as well as antimicrobial activity when Acetyl salicylic acid considered as standard.

| XXX | XXXI | XXXII | XXXIII |

R= OCH3, OH, CH3, Br, Cl

R1= H, Cl

A new series of 1-benzyl-5(3)-*p*-tolyl-1*H*-pyrazole-3(5)-carboxylic acid derivatives were prepared by (Caliskan et al.) All freshly prepared compounds were screened for their *in-vivo* analgesic and anti-inflammatory activities performed by *p*-benzoquinone- induced writhing test and the carrageenan-induced paw edema method. Among all prepared compounds, two compounds **XXXIV** and **XXXV** exhibited the best anti-inflammatory as well as analgesic activities [24].

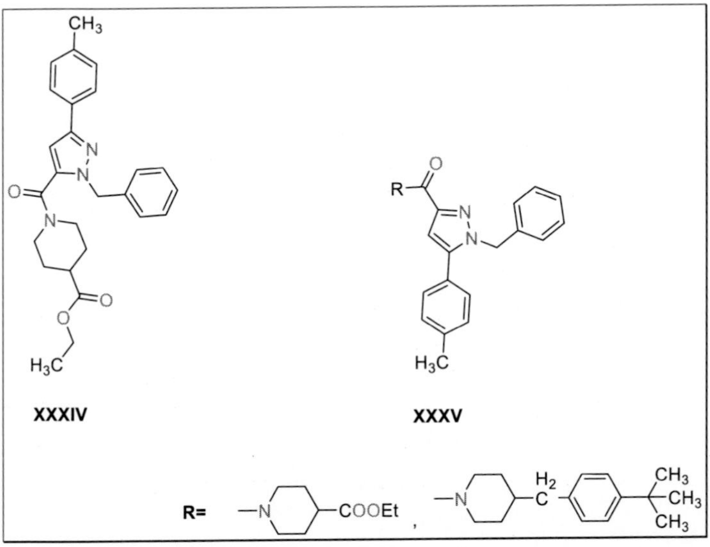

XXXIV

XXXV

R= —⟨N⟩—COOEt , —⟨N⟩—C(H₂)—⟨⟩—C(CH₃)(CH₃)CH₃

(Kalra et al.) introduced a novel series of 5-(Substituted-phenyl)-3-(furan-2-yl)-4,5-dihydro-1*H*-Pyrazole derivatives on treating hydrazine hydrate **(XXXVI)** with various chalcones **(XXXVII)**. All freshly prepared compounds were screened for their *in-vitro* anti-Inflammatory activity by using egg albumin method. Among to all synthesized products, an electron-releasing compound **XXXVIII** found to be the most potent candidate of this series with the IC_{50} value of 419.05 µg/ml when Diclofenac sodium used the standard drug [25].

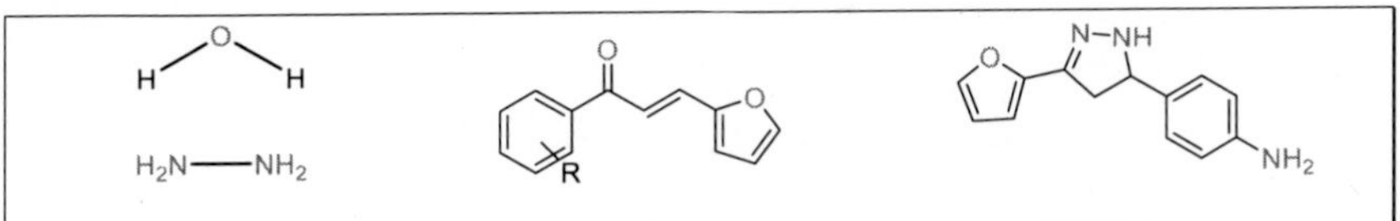

XXXVI   **XXXVII**   **XXXVIII**

R= 3',4'-OCH₃, 4-NO₂, 4-Br, 2',4'-OH, 4-OCH₃, 4-OH, 4-NH₂, 2-OH, 4-CH₃, 4-Cl, 2-Br-4-Cl, 2-Cl, 4-F, 2',4'-Cl

References

1. Bayly CI et al (1999) Structure-based design of COX-2 selectivity into flurbiprofen.Bioorganic & Medicinal Chemistry Letters 9 (3):307-312. DOI: 10.1016/s0960-894x(98)00717-3

2. Kurumbail RG et al (1997) Structural basis for selective inhibition of cyclooxygenase-2 by anti-inflammatory agents. Nature 84:644–648

3. Bakhle SY (1999) Structure of COX-1 and COX-2 enzymes and their interaction with inhibitors. Drugs Today 35(4-5):237. DOI: 10.1358/dot.1999.35.4-5.552200

4. Balsamo A et al (2004) Synthesis and COX-2 inhibitory properties of N-phenyl- and N-benzyl-substituted amides of 2-(4-methylsulfonylphenyl)cyclopent-1-ene-1-carboxylic acid and of their pyrazole, thiophene and isoxazole analogs. Farmaco 59 (1): 25-31. https://doi.org/10.1016/j.farmac.2003.09.003

5. Marnett LJ et al (2000) Biochemically based design of cyclooxygenase-2 (COX-2) inhibitors: Facile conversion of nonsteroidal antiinflammatory drugs to potent and highly selective COX-2 inhibitors. National Academy of Sciences 97(2):925-930; https://doi.org/10.1073/pnas.97.2.925

6. Fahmy H et al (2012) Synthesis and anti-inflammatory evaluation of new substituted 1-(3-chlorophenyl)-3-(4-methoxyphenyl)-1H-pyrazole derivatives. Acta Pol Pharm.69(3):411-21. PMID: 22594255

7. Rapposelli S et al (2004) Synthesis and COX-2 inhibitory properties of N-phenyl- and N-benzyl-substituted amides of 2-(4-methylsulfonylphenyl)cyclopent-1-ene-1-carboxylic acid and of their pyrazole, thiophene and isoxazole analogs. Farmaco (Societa Chimica Italiana) 59(1):25-31. DOI: 10.1016/j.farmac.2003.09.003

8. Abdellatif KRA et al (2015) Synthesis, cyclooxygenase inhibition, and anti-inflammatory evaluation of novel diarylheterocycles with a central pyrazole, pyrazoline, or pyridine ring. Med Chem Res. 24:2632. DOI: 10.1007/s00044-015-1327-7

9. Sahu SK et al (2008) Synthesis, Analgesic, Anti-inflammatory and Antimicrobial Activities of Some Novel Pyrazoline Derivatives. Tropical Journal of Pharmaceutical Research. 7(2):961-968. DOI: 10.4314/tjpr.v7i2.14664

10. Selvam TP et al (2014) Microwave-assisted synthesis, characterization and biological activity of novel pyrazole derivatives. Journal of Saudi Chemical Society. 18:1015–1021. http://dx.doi.org/10.1016/j.jscs.2011.12.006

11. Costa EA et al (2016) Design, synthesis and pharmacological evaluation of new anti-inflammatory compounds. European Journal of Pharmacology 791:195–204 http://dx.doi.org/10.1016/j.ejphar.2016.08.033

12. Lavanya P et al (2016) Synthesis and anti-inflammatory activity of some new 1,3,4-thiadiazoles containing pyrazole and pyrrole nucleus. Journal of Saudi Chemical Society 20:S306–S312. http://dx.doi.org/10.1016/j.jscs.2012.11.007

13. Mandour AH et al (2014) Synthesis, anti-inflammatory, analgesic and anticonvulsant activities of some new 4,6-dimethoxy-5-(heterocycles)benzofuran starting from naturally occurring visnagin. Arabian Journal of Chemistry 7:914–923. http://dx.doi.org/10.1016/j.arabjc.2012.12.041

14. Dhingra AK et al (2016) Synthesis and Anti-Inflammatory Activity of Some O-Propargylated-N-acetylpyrazole Derived from 1,3-Diarylpropenones. Hindawi Publishing Corporation International Journal of Medicinal Chemistry 2016 http://dx.doi.org/10.1155/2016/3156593

15. Kuo S et al (1984) Synthesis and Analgesic and Antiinflammatory Activities of 3,4-Dimethylpyrano[2,3-c]pyrazol-6-on Derivatives. J. Med. Chem. 27:539-544

16. Georgey H et al (2013) Synthesis of novel 1,3,4-trisubstituted pyrazoles as anti-inflammatory and analgesic agents. European Journal of Medicinal Chemistry 63:645-654. http://dx.doi.org/10.1016/j.ejmech.2013.03.005

17. Selvam TP et al (2012) Microwave-assisted synthesis, characterization and biological activity of novel pyrazole derivatives.Journal of Saudi Chemical Society 18:1015–1021. http://dx.doi.org/10.1016/j.jscs.2011.12.006

18. Kumar P et al (2012) Synthesis and biological evaluation of some pyrazole derivatives as anti-inflammatory–antibacterial agents. Med Chem Res 21:3396. https://doi.org/10.1007/s00044-011-9853-4

19. F Bakr et al (2012) Synthesis, antimicrobial, antioxidant, anti-inflammatory, and analgesic activities of some new 3-(20-thienyl)pyrazole-based heterocycles. Med Chem Res (2012) 21:1418–1426. DOI: 10.1007/s00044-011-9661-x

20. Domiati S et al (2016) Evaluation of anti-inflammatory, analgesic activities, and side effects of some pyrazole derivatives. Inflammopharmacology 24(4):163-72. DOI 10.1007/s10787-016-0270-7

21. Shchegol'kov EV et al (2006) Synthesis, analgesic and antipyretic activity of 2-(antipyrin-4-yl)hydrazones of 1,2,3-triketones and their derivatives. Pharmaceutical Chemistry Journal 40:27-29

37

22. M Nagwa et al (2012) Design and synthesis of some pyrazole derivatives of expected anti-inflammatory and analgesic activities. Med Chem Res 21:983–994. DOI: 10.1007/s00044-011-9606-4

23. Jayanna ND et al (2013) Synthesis, antimicrobial, analgesic activity, and molecular docking studies of novel 1-(5,7-dichloro-1,3-benzoxazol-2-yl)-3-phenyl-1Hpyrazole-4-carbaldehyde derivatives. Med Chem Res 22:5814. https://doi.org/10.1007/s00044-013-0565-9

24. Calıskan B et al (2013) Synthesis and evaluation of analgesic, anti-inflammatory, and anticancer activities of new pyrazole-3(5)-carboxylic acid derivatives. Med Chem Res 22:782–793 DOI: 10.1007/s00044-012-0072-4

25. Kalra R, Kumar S (2018) Anti-Inflammatory Activity of 5-(Substituted-Phenyl)-3-(Furan-2-Yl)-4,5-Dihydro-1h-Pyrazole Derivatives. Der Pharmacia Lettre 10(10):19-24

Chapter 5

Antimalarial Activity

Abstract The aim of this chapter is to provide focus on recent research work by various researchers on pyrazole derivatives which possessed significant antimalarial activity. There is a collection of literature work reported by various researchers on the antimalarial activity of pyrazole. Malaria is a disease which is borne through the bite of female *Anopheles* mosquito of genus Plasmodia parasites. The parasites of *Anopheles* mosquito start multiplying in the liver and latterly rupture the red blood cells.

Keywords Pyrazole, Heterocyclic, Antimalarial activity

Introduction

Malaria is a type of protozoan infection which is transmitted through the bite of female *Anopheles* mosquito (*eukaryotic* protozoan parasite) of genus *Plasmodia* and affect the red blood cells [1]. There are about 60 species of *Anopheles* mosquito which are existing worldwide and responsible for the transmission of malaria [2]. Childhood mortality increment was reported in the end of the 20th century [3]. Approximately, 3 billion people are possibility of malarial infection [4]. In 2016, more than 200 million cases were recorded [5]. In 1897, malaria cycle in mosquitoes (culicine) and birds infected with *Plasmodium relictum* was studied by Ronald Ross [6].

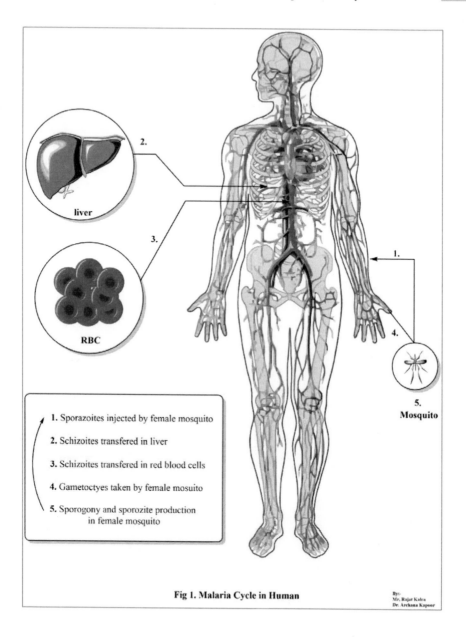

liver

RBC

2.

3.

1.

4.

5.
Mosquito

1. Sporazoites injected by female mosquito

2. Schizoites transfered in liver

3. Schizoites transfered in red blood cells

4. Gametoctyes taken by female mosuito

5. Sporogony and sporozite production
   in female mosquito

Fig 1. Malaria Cycle in Human

By:-
Mr. Rajat Kalra
Dr. Archana Kapoor

Antimalarial are the drugs which are used for the treatment and prevention of relapses of malaria. There are various mode of actions of antimalarial drugs such as *Tissue schizontocides, Hypnozoitocides, Blood schizontocides, Gametocytocides, Sporontocides* etc [7]. Pyrazole and its derivatives also possessed antimalarial activity [8-10]. In this chapter, there is a collection of literature work reported by various researchers on the antimalarial activity of pyrazole.

(Shaquiquzzaman et al.) prepared thirty-two novel pyrazole acrylic acid based oxadiazole and amide derivatives. All novel prepared derivatives were evaluated for their *in-vitro* antimalarial and anticancer activities by using the culture of chloroquine sensitive 3D7 strain of P. *falciparum*. Among the synthesized compounds, only four compounds found to be active but the compound **I** found to be most potent compound of this series with the IC_{50} value of 0.245 µg/mL. In conclusion, the compound **I** targeted an enzyme known as falcipain-2 and possessed antimalarial activity. Authors also noticed that cyclization (oxadiazole) recommended for antimalarial activity while non-cyclized compounds (amides) possessed anticancer activity [11].

I

Some novel aminomethylthiazole pyrazole carboxamide derivatives was prepared by (Chibale et al.) All newly prepared compounds were evaluated for their *in-vitro* antimalarial activity against K1, chloroquine resistant and chloroquine sensitive strains of P. *falciparum*. Among all reported compounds, compound **II** was found to be the most potent compound towards antiplasmodial activity against K1, chloroquine and multidrug resistant strain (with the IC_{50} value of 0.08 µM) and (IC_{50} value of 0.07 µM against NF54 chloroquine sensitive strain. It was also found that the compound **II** exhibited *invivo* antimalarial activity which was performed against the P. *berghei* in mouse model by the oral route. In conclusion, the compound **II** was found to be a lead compound and more work is required to reduce the hERG risk profile while improving the potency of the compound [12].

archanarajpal06@gmail.com
rohillarajat@gmail.com

41

II

A new series of some pyrazole derivatives were accomplished by (Bekhit et al.) All novel synthesized compounds were screened for their *in-vivo* anti-malarial activity against chloroquine sensitive strain of *P. berghei*. Further the most potent compounds were evaluated for their *in-vitro* antimalarial activity on chloroquine resistant (RKL9) strain of *P. falciparum*. In conclusion, among the synthesized compounds, compound **III** possessed the most potent antimalarial activity of this series with the IC$_{50}$ value of 0.033 ± 0.014 mM [13].

III

A new series of twenty pyraazole derivatives comparising pyrazole–pyrazoline nucleus hybrids with thioamide were synthesized by (Marella et al.) All newly reported compounds were screened for their *invitro* schizontocidal antimalarial activity towards CQ-sensitive 3D7 strain of *Plasmodium falciparum* and laterally the most active compounds were tested for their cytotoxicity effect towards VERO cell lines. During the quantitative structure–activity relationship (QSAR) study, it was found that the compound **IV** found to be the most active compound against *Plasmodium falciparum* with the IC$_{50}$ value of 1.13 μM [14].

IV

(Kumar et al.) reported novel pyrazole derivatives via condensation of 1,4-dihydropyridin- 4-yl-phenoxyacetohydrazides **(V)** with various substituted pyrazole carbaldehyde **(VI)**. All newly reported products were evaluated for their *in-vitro* antimalarial activity against *P. falciparum* at intra erythrocytic stage by using Schizonts maturation Inhibition (SMI) method. It was concluded that compound **VII** with the IC$_{50}$ value of 4.40 nM found to be four times more potent towards *P. falciparum* than the standard drug Chloroquine [15].

R= F, Cl, Me, H, Br, OMe, NO$_2$

A novel series of 1,5- and 1,3-diarylsubstituted pyrazoles derivatives were reported by (Surolia et al.) All newly synthesized compounds were tested for their antimalarial activity by using spectrophotometric assay method. It was noticed that the two compounds **VIII** (NAS-81) and **IX** (NAS-39) inhibited the enoyl-ACP reductase of *Plasmodium falciparum* with the IC$_{50}$ values of 30 μM and 50 μM [16].

Some new pyrazoles derivatives were reported by (Marella et al.) All newly synthesized compounds were tested for their *in-vitro* schizontocidal activity by using Trager and Jensen method. In conclusion, among the synthesized compounds, product **X** showed the most potent activity against CQ-sensitive 3D7 strain of *Plasmodium falciparum* with the IC$_{50}$ values of 31.13 μM [17].

X

References

1. Enna SJ and Bylund DB (Eds) (2008) xPharm: The Comprehensive Pharmacology Reference. Elsevier Inc. Isbn: 978-0-08-055232-3

2. Barrett ADT and Stanberry LR (2009) Vaccines for Biodefense and Emerging and Neglected Diseases. Academic Press. ISBN: 978-0-12-369408-9

3. Cohen J (Eds) et al (2017) Infectious Diseases. Elsevier. ISBN: 978-0-7020-6285-8

4. Magill AJ (Eds) et al (2012) Hunter's Tropical Medicine and Emerging Infectious Disease (9th Edn). Saunders, Elsevier Inc. ISBN: 978-1-4160-4390-4

5. Ashley Elizabeth A et al (2018) Malaria. Lancet (London, England) 391(10130):1608-1621. https://doi.org/10.1016/S0140-6736(18)30324-6

6. Cox FE (2010) History of the discovery of the malaria parasites and their vectors. Parasites Vectors 3:5. https://doi.org/10.1186/1756-3305-3-5

7. Warhurst DC (1987) Antimalarial Drugs. Drugs 33:50. https://doi.org/10.2165/00003495-198733010-00003

8. N Jose et al (2002) Synthesis and Antimalarial Activity of Substituted Pyrazole Derivatives. Arzneimittelforschung 52(6):482-488. DOI: 10.1055/s-0031-1299918

9. Tabassum K et al (2018) Imidazole and Pyrazole: Privileged Scaffolds for Anti-Infective Activity. Bentham 15(6):459-475. DOI: 10.2174/1570193X15666171211170100

10. Shilpy A et al (2018) Pyrazole Schiff Base Hybrids as Anti-Malarial Agents: Synthesis, In Vitro Screening and Computational Study. Bentham 21:194-203. https://doi.org/10.2174/1386207321666180213092911

11. Shaquiquzzaman M et al (2018) Synthesis of pyrazole acrylic acid based oxadiazole and amide derivatives as antimalarial and anticancer agents. Bioorganic Chemistry 77:106–124. https://doi.org/10.1016/j.bioorg.2018.01.007

12. Chibale K et al (2011) Novel Orally Active Antimalarial Thiazoles. J. Med. Chem 54:7713–7719. dx.doi.org/10.1021/jm201108k

13. Bekhi AA et al (2012) Synthesis and Biological Evaluation of Some Pyrazole Derivatives as Anti-Malarial Agents. Arch. Pharm. Chem. Life Sci 345:147–154. DOI: 10.1002/ardp.201100078

14. Marella A et al (2015) Novel pyrazole–pyrazoline hybrids endowed with thioamide as antimalarial agents: their synthesis and 3D-QSAR studies, Journal of Enzyme Inhibition and Medicinal Chemistry 30:(4):597-606. https://doi.org/10.3109/14756366.2014.958081

15. Kumar P et al (2017) Design, synthesis, conformational and molecular docking study of some novel acyl hydrazone based molecular hybrids as antimalarial and antimicrobial agents. Chemistry Central Journal 11:115. DOI: 10.1186/s13065-017-0344-7

16. Surolia N et al (2006) Synthesis and Evaluation of Substituted Pyrazoles: Potential Antimalarials Targeting the Enoyl-ACP Reductase of Plasmodium Falciparum. Synthetic Communications 36:(2):215-226. DOI: 10.1080/00397910500334561

17. Marella A et al (2014) Novel pyrazole–pyrazoline hybrids endowed with thioamide as antimalarial agents: their synthesis and 3D-QSAR studies. J Enzyme Inhib Med Chem, Early Online: 1–10. DOI: 10.3109/14756366.2014.958081

Chapter 6

Antiviral Activity

Abstract The aim of this chapter is to provide focus on recent research work carried out by various researchers on pyrazole derivatives which possessed significant antiviral activity. Viral is disease which is caused by virus. They have capability to multiply and produce viruses like themselves. Pyrazole derivatives possessed antiviral activity which uses for in the treatment of viral infection of various types.

Keywords Pyrazole, Antiviral activity

Introduction

Antiviral drugs are those which are used to treat the specific viral infection. A virus is formed by an organization of macromolecules. The vital assumption regarding viral pathogenesis is that they transfer from cell to cell. The virus consists of **(i)** The capsid (outermost shell which cover the nucleic acid), **(ii)** The nucleocapsid (a type of protein shell), **(iii)** The envelope (also known as virus membrane, this is a lipid bilayer), and **(iv)** The core (a shell which cover protein shell). There are two types of viral nucleic acid **(i)**RNA Viruses and **(ii)** DNA Viruses [1]. [Perspectives in Medical Virology Elisver]

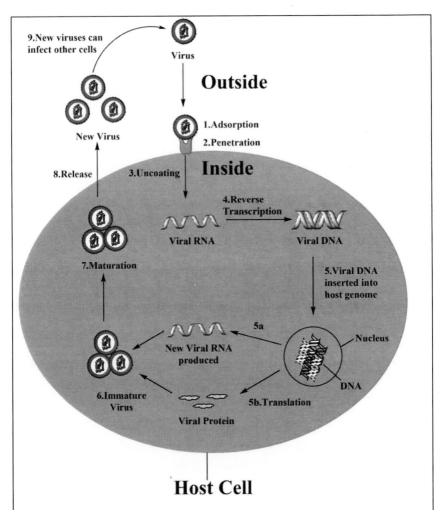

Fig.1 General Virus Life Cycle. **1** Adsorption. In this step virus directly attached to the host recptors. **2** Pentration. Now the virus enter into the host cell. **3** Uncoating. The covering of virus (capsid) remains outside the host cell and the genatic material of virus is entered into host body. **4** Reverse Transcripition. Production of new viral DNA from viral genome. **5a** Multipal viral genome now copy with host DNA machinery. **5b** The viral genome enter into cytoplasm of cell or into nucleoplasma and further produce new viral protein. **6** Immature Virus. New viral genomes and the viral protein are assembles into capsid. **7** Maturation. New copies of virus completely produced and ready to rupture the host cell. **8** Release. The mature virus released outside from the host cell and repeat of this cycle, in new host cell.

By:-
Mr. Rajat Kalra
Dr. Archana Kapoor

Pyrazole and its derivatives possess antiviral activity [2]. In this chapter, there is a collection of literature work reported by various researchers on the antiviral activity of pyrazole.

A new series of 3-((2-((1E,4E)-3-oxo-5-arylpenta-1,4-dien-1-yl)phenoxy)methyl)-4(3*H*)-quinazolinone derivatives were introduced by (Song et al.) All nwly prepared compounds were screened for their antiviral bioassay on tobacco mosaic virus (TMV). In conclusion, among the synthesized products, the compound **I** was found to be the most active compound of this series when compared to standard drug Ningnanmycin [3].

I

R₁= H, 8-CH₃   **R₂= 2-OCH₃Phenyl, 2-thiophenyl,**   **X= 2-O, 4-O**
                   3,4-di-OCH₃phenyl, 4-OCH₃phenyl

(Song et al.) again reported a novel series of pyrazole derivatives via reaction of 1-substituted phenyl-3-methyl-5-substituted phenylthio-4-pyrazolaldoximes **(II)** with chloromethylated heterocyclic compounds **(III)**. All newly synthesized products were evalvated for their antiviral activity and the results suggested that the compound **(IV)** exhibited the most promising antiviral activity against the TMV with the EC₅₀ values of 58.7 and 65.3 µg/mL when Ningnanmycin used as the standard drug [4].

II   **III**   **IV**

R₁= H, 4Cl   **R₂= Me, F**   **R₃=**

(El-Sabbagh et al.) reported a novel series of pyrazole and thiazole derivatives via taking α, β-unsaturated ketones as stating material. All newly reported compounds were screened for their

49

antiviral activity against vaccinia virus (Lederle strain) and found that compound **(V)** showed the most potent activity against the vaccinia virus (Lederle strain) in HEL cell cultures with EC_{50} value of 7μg/ml when Ribavirin considered as the standard drug [5].

V

Again a novel series of N-phenylpyrazoles and dihydroisoxazles via taking α, β-unsaturated ketones as staring material was prepared by (Rashad et al.). All newly synthesized candidates were evalvated for their antiviral bioassay against hepatitis A virus and herpes simplex virus type 1. In conclusion, among the synthesized products, candidate **VI** found to be the most potent of this series [6].

VI

R= Cl, CH$_3$

A novel compound named BPR1P0034 **(VII)** with the effective activity against anti-influenza virus was discovered by (Shih et al.) BPR1P0034 is the first pyrazole-based anti-influenza compound ever discovered. During the SAR study, it was found that more lead compounds can be synthesized by changing the hydrazone part of BPR1P0034 structure. During plaque reduction assay, it was found that the effective 50% inhibitory concentration (IC_{50}) values of BPR1P0034 was 0.42 ± 0.11 μM [7].

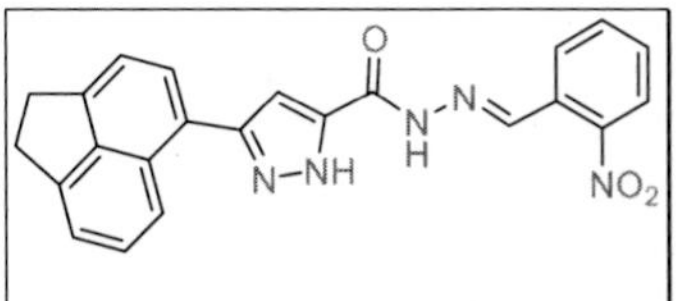

VII

BPR1P0034

(Tantawy et al.) produced the novel series of 3-methyl-1,5-diphenyl-1*H*-pyrazole derivatives via the reaction of 3-methyl-1,5-diphenyl-1*H*-pyrazole-4-carbaldehyde **(VIII)** with various acetophenones **(IX)** through the Claisen-Schmidt condensation. All newly prepared products were screened for their *in vitro* antiviral activity against herpes simplex virus type-1. In conclusion, among the synthesized compounds, four compounds **X, XI, XII** and **XIII** were found to be the most potent antiviral against when compared to standard drug Acyclovir [8].

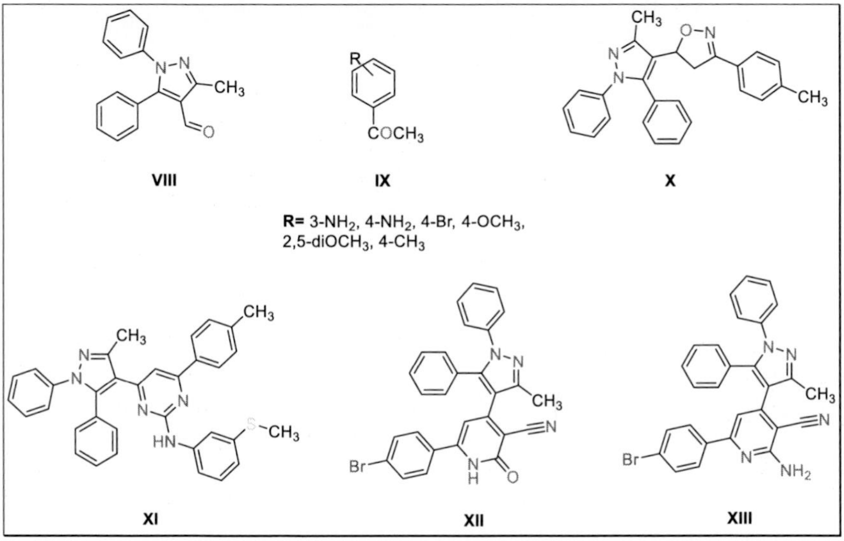

VIII   **IX**   **X**

R= 3-NH$_2$, 4-NH$_2$, 4-Br, 4-OCH$_3$,
2,5-diOCH$_3$, 4-CH$_3$

XI   **XII**   **XIII**

Some novel pyrazole and isoxazole based heterocycles was synthesized by (Dawood et al.) All novel synthesized compounds were evaluated for their antiviral activity. It was found that the compound **XIV** possessed the most effective activity against the Herpes simplex type-1 (HSV-1) and decreased the number of viral plaques by 69% [9].

51

XIV

References

1. Mateu Mg (Ed) (2013) Structure and Physics of Viruses: An Integrated Textbook. Springer Science+Business Media Dordrecht. ISBN 978-94-007-6551-1. DOI: 10.1007/978-94-007-6552-8

2. I.El-Sabbagh OI et al (2009) Synthesis and antiviral activity of new pyrazole and thiazole derivatives. European Journal of Medicinal Chemistry 44(9):3746-3753. https://doi.org/10.1016/j.ejmech.2009.03.038

3. Song B et al (2014) Synthesis and Antiviral Bioactivity of Novel 3-((2-(((1E,4E)-3-Oxo-5-arylpenta-1,4-dien-1-yl)phenoxy)methyl)-4(3H)-quinazolinone Derivatives. American Chemical Society J. Agric. Food Chem 62(36):8928–8934. dx.doi.org/10.1021/jf502162y

4. Song BA et al (2008) Synthesis and Antiviral Activities of Pyrazole Derivatives Containing an Oxime Moiety. J. Agric. Food Chem 56:10160–10167. DOI: 10.1021/jf802489e

5. El-Sabbagh O et al (2009) Synthesis and antiviral activity of new pyrazole and thiazole derivatives. European Journal of Medicinal Chemistry 44:3746–3753. DOI: 10.1016/j.ejmech.2009.03.038

6. Rashad AA et al (2010) Design, synthesis and preliminary antiviral screening of new N-phenylpyrazole and dihydroisoxazole derivatives. Med Chem Res 19:1025–1035 DOI: 10.1007/s00044-009-9248-y

7. Shih SR et al (2010) RPeyserarachzole compound BPR1P0034 with potent and selective anti-influenza virus activity. Journal of Biomedical Science 17:13.

8. Tantawy AS et al (2012) Synthesis and antiviral activity of new 3-methyl-1,5-diphenyl-1Hpyrazole derivatives. Med Chem Res 21:4139–4149. DOI: 10.1007/s00044-011-9960-2

9. Dawood KM (2011) Synthesis, anti-HSV-1, and cytotoxic activities of some new pyrazole- and isoxazole-based heterocycles. Med Chem Res 20:912–919. DOI: 10.1007/s00044-010-9420-4

Chapter 7

Market Drug Containing Pyrazole Moiety

Abstract In this chapter there is some collection of drugs containing pyrazole nucleus which are available in the market. These drugs possess various different activities such as gastric secretory, analgesic and antipyretic, arthritis, acute pain, osteoarthritis, painful menstruation, NSAID, broad spectrum insecticide, antidote, antipsychotic effects, anticancer, improves long term memory acquisition, anxiety neuroses etc.

Keywords Pyrazole, Market drug, NSAID, anxiety neuros

List of market drug which containing Pyrazole moiety

1. Betazole
2. Phenazone (INN)
3. Celecoxib
4. Lonazolac
5. Tepoxalin
6. Fipronil
7. Fomepizole
8. CDPPB
9. Crizotinib
10. AS-19
11. Psigodal

1. Betazole

IUPAC Name: 2-(1*H*-pyrazol-5-yl)ethanamine

Molecular Weight: 111.148 g/mol

Molecular Formula: $C_5H_9N_3$

Use: Clinically tested for gastric secretory

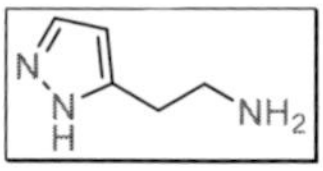

2. Phenazone(INN)

IUPAC Name: 1,5-dimethyl-2-phenylpyrazol-3-one

Molecular Formula: $C_{11}H_{12}N_2O$

Molecular Weight: 188.23 g/mol

Use: Analgesic and Antipyretic

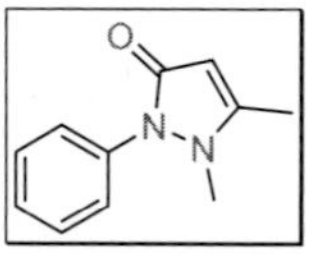

3. Celecoxib

IUPAC Name: 4-[5-(4-methylphenyl)-3-(trifluoromethyl)pyrazol-1-yl]benzenesulfonamide

Molecular Formula: $C_{17}H_{14}F_3N_3O_2S$

Molecular Weight: 381.373 g/mol

Use: (NSAID) Treatment of rheumatoid arthritis, acute pain, osteoarthritis, painful menstruation and menstrual symptoms.

4. Lonazolac

IUPAC Name: 2-[3-(4-chlorophenyl)-1-phenylpyrazol-4-yl]acetic acid

Molecular Formula: $C_{17}H_{13}ClN_2O_2$

Molecular Weight: 312.753 g/mol

Use: Used as NSAID

5. Tepoxalin

IUPAC Name: 3-(5-(4-chlorophenyl)-1-(4-methoxyphenyl)-1H-pyrazol-3-yl)-N-hydroxy-N-methylpropanamide

Molecular Formula: $C_{20}H_{20}ClN_3O_3$

Molecular Weight: 385.848 g/mol

Use: Non-steroidal antiinflammatory drug apporved in USA and the European Union used for veterinary.

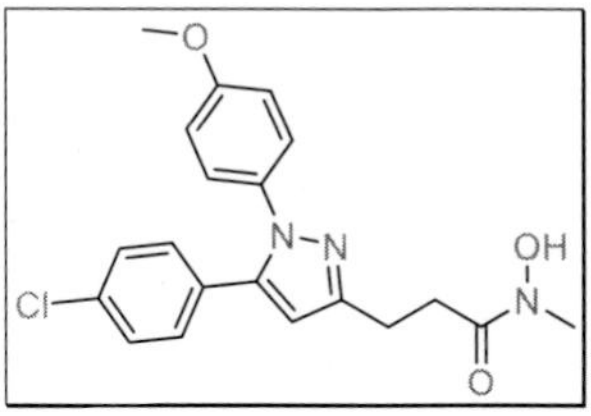

6. Fipronil

IUPAC Name: 5-amino-1-[2,6-dichloro-4-(trifluoromethyl)phenyl]-4 (trifluoromethylsulfinyl)pyrazole-3-carbonitrile

Molecular Formula: $C_{12}H_4Cl_2F_6N_4OS$

Molecular Weight: 437.141 g/mol

Use: Broad spectrum insecticide by blocking the passage of chloride ions through the GABA receptor and glutamate-gated chloride channels (Glu Cl) and effect on CNS of insect

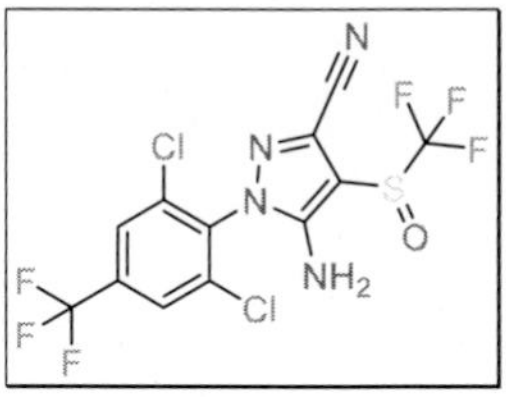

7. Fomepizole

IUPAC Name: 4-methyl-1*H*-pyrazole

Molecular Formula: $C_4H_6N_2$

Molecular Weight: 82.106 g/mol

Use: Antidote for confirmed or suspected methanol or ethylene glycol poisoning

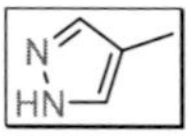

57

8. CDPPB

Molecular Formula: $C_{23}H_{16}N_4O$

Molecular Weight: 364.408 g/mol

IUPAC Name: 3-cyano-N-(1,3-diphenyl-1H-pyrazol-5-yl)benzamide

Use: Antipsychotic effects in animal models

9. Crizotinib

IUPAC Name: 3-[(1~{R})-1-(2,6-dichloro-3-fluorophenyl)ethoxy]-5-(1-piperidin-4-ylpyrazol-4-yl)pyridin-2-amine

Molecular Formula: $C_{21}H_{22}Cl_2FN_5O$

Molecular Weight: 450.339 g/mol

Use: Treatment of cancer (anticancer) inhibitor of (anaplasticlymphomakinase) and ROS-1

10. AS-19

IUPAC Name: (2S)-N,N-dimethyl-5-(1,3,5-trimethylpyrazol-4-yl)-1,2,3,4-tetrahydronaphthalen-2-amine

Molecular Formula: $C_{18}H_{25}N_3$

Molecular Weight: 283.419 g/mol

Use: Improves long term memory acquisition. Potent agonist of 5HT-7 receptor.

11. Psigodal

IUPAC Name: 1-(3-chlorophenyl)-4-[2-(5-methyl-1*H*-pyrazol-3-yl)ethyl]piperazine

Molecular Formula: C16H21ClN4

Molecular Weight: 304.822 g/mol

Use: Treatment of anxiety neuroses.

References

1. Yerragunta V et al (2014) Pyrazole and Its Biological Activity. PharmaTutor 2(1)40-48

2. National Center for Biotechnology Information. PubChem Compound Database; CID=7741, https://pubchem.ncbi.nlm.nih.gov/compound/7741 (accessed Feb. 4, 2019)

3. National Center for Biotechnology Information. PubChem Compound Database; CID=2206, https://pubchem.ncbi.nlm.nih.gov/compound/2206 (accessed Feb. 4, 2019)

4. National Center for Biotechnology Information. PubChem Compound Database; CID=2662, https://pubchem.ncbi.nlm.nih.gov/compound/2662 (accessed Feb. 4, 2019)

5. National Center for Biotechnology Information. PubChem Compound Database; CID=68706, https://pubchem.ncbi.nlm.nih.gov/compound/68706 (accessed Feb. 4, 2019)

6. National Center for Biotechnology Information. PubChem Compound Database; CID=59757, https://pubchem.ncbi.nlm.nih.gov/compound/59757 (accessed Feb. 4, 2019)

7. National Center for Biotechnology Information. PubChem Compound Database; CID=3352, https://pubchem.ncbi.nlm.nih.gov/compound/3352 (accessed Feb. 4, 2019)

8. National Center for Biotechnology Information. PubChem Compound Database; CID=3406, https://pubchem.ncbi.nlm.nih.gov/compound/3406 (accessed Feb. 4, 2019)

9. National Center for Biotechnology Information. PubChem Compound Database; CID=11245456, https://pubchem.ncbi.nlm.nih.gov/compound/11245456 (accessed Feb. 4, 2019)

10. National Center for Biotechnology Information. PubChem Compound Database; CID=11626560, https://pubchem.ncbi.nlm.nih.gov/compound/11626560 (accessed Feb. 4, 2019)

11. National Center for Biotechnology Information. PubChem Compound Database; CID=23642275, https://pubchem.ncbi.nlm.nih.gov/compound/23642275 (accessed Feb. 4, 2019)

12. National Center for Biotechnology Information. PubChem Compound Database; CID=71897, https://pubchem.ncbi.nlm.nih.gov/compound/71897 (accessed Feb. 4, 2019)

13. Kalra R, Kumar S (2018) Valuable Heterocyclic Pyrazole. Lambert Academic Publishing

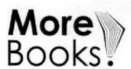
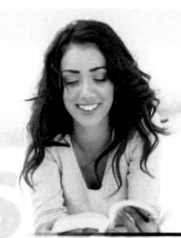 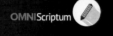

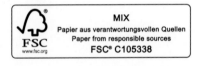

Printed by Books on Demand GmbH, Norderstedt / Germany